FATTY LIVER DIET COOKBOOK FOR SENIORS

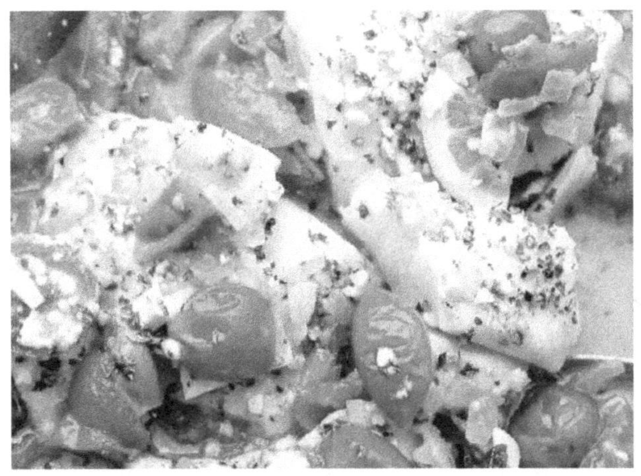

The Ultimate Guide to Easy and Delicious Weight Loss Recipes to Detoxify and Revitalize Your Liver, With 30 Day Meal Plan.

Joshua S. Gray

Table of Contents

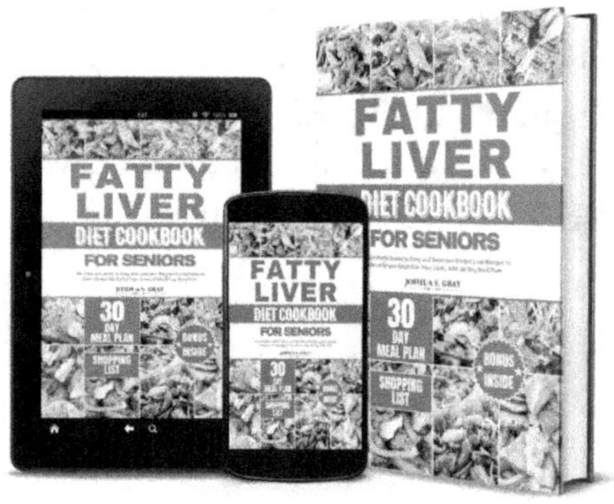

How to Use This Book

Introduction: Begin by reading the introduction to understand the purpose of this cookbook. Fatty liver disease, the importance of managing fatty liver disease through diet, lifestyle changes, weight control and lots more.

Recipe Sections: Explore the different sections of the cookbook, including breakfast, lunch, dinner, snacks, and desserts. Each section contains a variety of delicious and nutritious recipes tailored to support liver health and promote overall well-being.

Meal Plans: Utilize the 30-day meal plan provided in the cookbook to help you plan your meals and stay on track with your dietary goals. This meal plan offers a balanced approach to eating, ensuring you get the nutrients you need while managing fatty liver disease.

Nutritional Information: Pay attention to the nutritional information provided for each recipe, including calories, protein, fat, and carbohydrates. This information will help you make informed choices about your meals and monitor your intake as part of your overall dietary plan.

Meal Planner Journal: Use the meal planner journal included in the cookbook to track your meals, snacks, and overall dietary intake. This journal can help you stay organized, identify patterns in your eating habits, and make adjustments as needed to support your health goals.

Shopping List: Refer to the shopping list section to ensure you have all the necessary ingredients on hand before you start cooking. Having a well-stocked pantry and fridge makes it easier to prepare healthy meals at home and reduces the temptation to eat unhealthy convenience foods.

Weight Loss Exercises for Seniors: Discover a selection of low-impact exercises tailored for seniors to complement your dietary journey. These exercises promote weight loss, improve cardiovascular health, and enhance overall fitness, helping you achieve your health goals more effectively.

Notes/Progress Report: Take advantage of the notes and progress report section to jot down any observations, reflections, or goals related to your dietary and exercise journey. Keeping track of your progress can help you stay motivated and focused on achieving your health goals.

Remember that taking control of your health is a proactive decision. By using this cookbook, incorporating exercise into your routine, and making positive changes to your lifestyle, you're investing in a healthier and happier future.

INTRODUCTION

Have you ever wondered why some decisions you make that seem healthy may actually be negatively affecting the health of your liver as you age? Imagine that after a long and happy life, you are suddenly told that you have fatty liver disease. You may believe that eliminating all fats from your diet is the best course of action, or you may consider taking drastic methods to lose the extra weight. But what if I told you that there may be more harm than good associated with these widespread misconceptions regarding the treatment of fatty liver disease in seniors?

Millions of elderly people worldwide suffer from fatty liver disease, a disorder marked by an accumulation of fat in the liver cells.

Non-alcoholic fatty liver disease (NAFLD) is becoming more common in older adults, despite being frequently linked to excessive alcohol consumption. This is because of factors like obesity, insulin resistance, and metabolic syndrome.

But do not worry—help is at hand. You'll discover a wealth of information in this Fatty Liver Diet Cookbook for Seniors that is especially designed to address the special dietary requirements of senior citizens. This cookbook is your go-to resource for managing fatty liver disease and regaining your energy. It includes delicious and liver-friendly recipes as well as insightful advice on choosing healthier foods.

On your path to improved liver health, let this cookbook serve as your guiding light. Embrace the empowering knowledge that is waiting for you within these pages and bid farewell to confusion and frustration. One healthy meal at a time, together, we'll navigate the route to wellbeing.

CHAPTER 1

What is Fatty Liver Disease

Fatty liver disease, also known as hepatic steatosis, is a condition characterized by the accumulation of excess fat in the liver cells. This build-up of fat can interfere with the liver's normal function and lead to inflammation and liver damage over time. Fatty liver disease is commonly associated with alcohol consumption, but it can also occur in individuals who do not consume excessive amounts of alcohol, a condition known as non-alcoholic fatty liver disease (NAFLD).

There are two main types of fatty liver disease:

1.   Alcoholic Fatty Liver Disease (AFLD): This type of fatty liver disease is caused by excessive alcohol consumption. Chronic alcohol abuse can lead to the accumulation of fat in the liver cells, which can eventually progress to inflammation and liver damage.

2.   Non-Alcoholic Fatty Liver Disease (NAFLD): NAFLD is the most common form of fatty liver disease and occurs in individuals who do not consume significant amounts of alcohol. It is often associated with obesity, insulin resistance, type 2 diabetes, high cholesterol, and metabolic syndrome. NAFLD encompasses a spectrum of conditions ranging from simple fatty liver (steatosis) to non-alcoholic steatohepatitis (NASH), which involves inflammation and liver cell damage, and may progress to more severe liver complications such as cirrhosis and liver cancer.

Fatty liver disease can be asymptomatic in its early stages, but as it progresses, individuals may experience symptoms such as fatigue, abdominal discomfort, and liver enlargement. Early detection and management of fatty liver disease are crucial to prevent complications and preserve liver health. Lifestyle modifications such as adopting a healthy diet, maintaining a healthy weight, exercising regularly, limiting alcohol consumption, and managing underlying medical conditions are key components of treatment for fatty liver disease. Regular medical monitoring and consultation with a healthcare provider are also essential for managing the condition effectively.

Causes of Fatty Liver Disease

Fatty liver disease, also known as hepatic steatosis, can develop due to various factors, including lifestyle choices, medical conditions, and genetic predispositions. Here are some of the primary causes of fatty liver disease:

1. **Alcohol Consumption:** Excessive alcohol consumption is one of the leading causes of fatty liver disease. Chronic alcohol abuse can lead to the accumulation of fat in the liver cells, impairing liver function and potentially causing inflammation and liver damage. Alcoholic fatty liver disease (AFLD) ranges from simple fatty liver to more severe conditions like alcoholic hepatitis and cirrhosis.

2.   **Obesity and Metabolic Syndrome:** Non-alcoholic fatty liver disease (NAFLD) is closely associated with obesity and metabolic syndrome, which includes conditions such as insulin resistance, type 2 diabetes, high blood pressure, and abnormal lipid levels. Excess body weight, particularly visceral adipose tissue (fat around the abdomen), increases the risk of fat accumulation in the liver cells.

3.   **Insulin Resistance:** Insulin resistance, a condition in which the body's cells become resistant to the effects of insulin, can contribute to the development of fatty liver disease. When insulin resistance occurs, the liver produces more glucose and triglycerides, contributing to fat accumulation in the liver.

4.   **Dietary Factors:** Consuming a diet high in unhealthy fats, sugars, and refined carbohydrates can increase the risk of fatty liver

disease. Diets high in processed foods, sugary beverages, and fried foods can contribute to weight gain and metabolic disturbances, promoting fat accumulation in the liver.

5. **Medications:** Certain medications, including corticosteroids, tamoxifen, methotrexate, and some antiretroviral drugs, can cause or exacerbate fatty liver disease. These medications may disrupt lipid metabolism or impair liver function, leading to fat accumulation in the liver cells.

6. **Genetic Factors:** Genetic predisposition may also play a role in the development of fatty liver disease. Some individuals may have genetic variations that increase their susceptibility to fat accumulation in the liver or impair their ability to metabolize fats effectively.

7.   **Other Factors:** Other factors such as rapid weight loss, malnutrition, viral hepatitis (such as hepatitis C), and certain inherited metabolic disorders can also contribute to the development of fatty liver disease.

Understanding the underlying causes of fatty liver disease is essential for prevention, early detection, and management. Lifestyle modifications, including maintaining a healthy weight, adopting a balanced diet, regular exercise, limiting alcohol consumption, and managing underlying medical conditions, are key strategies for preventing and managing fatty liver disease. It's important for individuals at risk or diagnosed with fatty liver disease to work closely with healthcare professionals to develop personalized treatment plans and minimize the risk of complications.

Managing Fatty Liver Through Diet

Managing fatty liver disease through diet is crucial for improving liver health, reducing inflammation, and preventing disease progression. Here are some dietary strategies to help manage fatty liver disease effectively:

1.   **Follow a Balanced Diet:** Adopting a balanced and nutritious diet is essential for managing fatty liver disease. Eat a range of whole foods, such as fruits, vegetables, whole grains, lean meats, and healthy fats. Limit your intake of processed foods, sugary snacks, and foods high in saturated and trans fats.

2.   **Choose Healthy Fats:** Incorporate healthy fats into your diet, such as omega-3 fatty acids found in fatty fish (salmon, mackerel, sardines), flaxseeds, chia seeds, and

walnuts. These fats have anti-inflammatory properties and can help reduce liver inflammation. Additionally, use heart-healthy oils like olive oil, avocado oil, and flaxseed oil for cooking and salad dressings.

3. **Limit Saturated and Trans Fats:** Reduce your intake of saturated and trans fats, which can contribute to liver inflammation and worsen fatty liver disease. Avoid fried foods, processed meats, full-fat dairy products, and commercially baked goods, which are high in these unhealthy fats.

4. **Control Portion Sizes:** Be mindful of portion sizes to avoid overeating and promote weight management. Opt for smaller portions of high-calorie foods and fill up on nutrient-dense foods like fruits, vegetables, and lean proteins.

5.   **Monitor Carbohydrate Intake:** Limit your intake of refined carbohydrates and added sugars, as they can contribute to insulin resistance and fat accumulation in the liver. Choose whole grains, fruits, and vegetables as sources of carbohydrates, and minimize consumption of sugary snacks, desserts, and beverages.

6.   **Increase Fiber Intake:** Fiber-rich foods help promote digestion, regulate blood sugar levels, and support healthy weight management. Include plenty of fiber-rich foods in your diet, such as fruits, vegetables, whole grains, legumes, and nuts.

7.   **Stay Hydrated:** Drink plenty of water throughout the day to stay hydrated and support liver function. Limit consumption of sugary beverages, alcohol, and caffeinated drinks, as

they can contribute to dehydration and liver damage.

8.   **Moderate Alcohol Consumption:** If you have fatty liver disease, it's important to limit or avoid alcohol altogether. Even moderate alcohol consumption can worsen liver inflammation and contribute to disease progression.

9.   **Seek Professional Guidance:** Consult with a registered dietitian or healthcare provider for personalized dietary recommendations tailored to your specific needs and medical history. They can help you create a customized meal plan and provide ongoing support to help you manage fatty liver disease effectively.

By making informed dietary choices and adopting a healthy lifestyle, you can significantly improve liver health, reduce inflammation, and better manage fatty liver disease. Remember to prioritize whole, nutrient-rich foods, limit unhealthy fats and sugars, and seek professional guidance for personalized dietary recommendations. With dedication and consistency, you can take control of your health and support your liver's well-being.

CHAPTER 2

Importance of Diet and Nutrition in Fatty Liver Disease

Diet and nutrition play a critical role in the development, progression, and management of fatty liver disease. Here's why they are important:

1.   **Fat Accumulation:** Fatty liver disease is characterized by the accumulation of fat in the liver cells. Diet directly influences the amount and type of fat stored in the liver. Consuming a diet high in unhealthy fats, sugars, and refined carbohydrates can contribute to fat accumulation in the liver, exacerbating the condition.

2. **Liver Inflammation:** A poor diet high in processed foods, sugary beverages, and unhealthy fats can promote inflammation in the liver. Inflammation exacerbates liver damage and contributes to the progression of fatty liver disease. On the other hand, consuming a diet rich in anti-inflammatory foods, such as fruits, vegetables, and omega-3 fatty acids, can help reduce inflammation and protect liver health.

3. **Insulin Resistance:** Insulin resistance, a condition in which the body's cells become resistant to the effects of insulin, is closely linked to fatty liver disease. A diet high in refined carbohydrates and added sugars can contribute to insulin resistance, leading to increased fat accumulation in the liver. Adopting a diet that promotes stable blood sugar levels and insulin sensitivity can help prevent and manage insulin resistance and fatty liver disease.

4.   **Weight Management:** Obesity and excess body weight are major risk factors for fatty liver disease. Diet plays a central role in weight management, as both the quantity and quality of food consumed impact overall energy balance. Adopting a balanced diet that supports healthy weight loss or weight maintenance is essential for managing fatty liver disease and reducing liver fat accumulation.

5.   **Nutrient Intake:** Fatty liver disease can affect nutrient absorption and metabolism in the body. It's important for individuals with fatty liver disease to consume a nutrient-rich diet that provides essential vitamins, minerals, antioxidants, and other nutrients needed for liver health and overall well-being. Nutrient deficiencies can exacerbate liver damage and impair liver function.

6. **Alcohol Consumption:** For individuals with alcoholic fatty liver disease (AFLD), limiting or abstaining from alcohol consumption is essential for managing the condition. Alcohol can exacerbate liver inflammation and damage, worsening fatty liver disease and increasing the risk of complications such as cirrhosis and liver cancer.

Adopting a healthy diet that is rich in whole foods, low in unhealthy fats and sugars, and supports weight management and liver health is essential for preventing and managing fatty liver disease.

Weight Control and Fatty Liver

Weight control plays a crucial role in the management of fatty liver disease. Excess body weight, particularly abdominal obesity, is a significant risk factor for the development and progression of fatty liver disease. Here's how weight control impacts fatty liver:

1.   **Reducing Liver Fat Accumulation:** Excess body weight, especially visceral adipose tissue (fat around the abdomen), is closely associated with fat accumulation in the liver. Losing weight can help reduce liver fat content and improve liver function. Even modest weight loss of 5-10% of total body weight has been shown to significantly decrease liver fat content and improve liver health in individuals with fatty liver disease.

2.   **Improving Insulin Sensitivity:** Obesity and insulin resistance often go hand in hand, contributing to the development and progression of fatty liver disease. Insulin resistance impairs the body's ability to regulate blood sugar levels and promotes fat accumulation in the liver. By promoting weight loss and improving insulin sensitivity, individuals with fatty liver disease can reduce the risk of further liver damage and complications.

3.   **Decreasing Inflammation:** Obesity is associated with chronic low-grade inflammation, which can exacerbate liver inflammation and contribute to liver damage in individuals with fatty liver disease. Losing weight can help reduce inflammation throughout the body, including in the liver,

thereby improving liver function and reducing the risk of disease progression.

4. **Lowering Risk of Complications:** Fatty liver disease is associated with an increased risk of developing serious complications such as liver fibrosis, cirrhosis, and liver cancer. Obesity and excess body weight further elevate the risk of these complications. By achieving and maintaining a healthy weight, individuals with fatty liver disease can lower their risk of developing advanced liver disease and associated complications.

5. **Promoting Overall Health:** In addition to its impact on liver health, weight control has numerous benefits for overall health and well-being. Losing weight can improve cardiovascular health, reduce the risk of type 2 diabetes, lower blood pressure, and improve mobility and quality of life.

Weight control is a cornerstone of fatty liver disease management. Adopting healthy lifestyle habits such as following a balanced diet, engaging in regular physical activity, and maintaining a healthy weight can significantly improve liver health and reduce the risk of complications associated with fatty liver disease.

CHAPTER 3

Shopping List

Creating a shopping list tailored to a fatty liver diet involves selecting nutrient-rich foods that support liver health while minimizing consumption of unhealthy fats, sugars, and processed foods. Here's a comprehensive shopping list for individuals with fatty liver disease:

Proteins:

- Lean cuts of poultry (skinless chicken breasts, turkey breast)
- Fish rich in omega-3 fatty acids (salmon, mackerel, sardines)
- Lean cuts of beef (sirloin, tenderloin)
- Eggs

- Tofu

- Low-fat dairy products (skim milk, low-fat yogurt, cottage cheese)

- Legumes (lentils, chickpeas, black beans)

Fruits:

- Berries (blueberries, strawberries, raspberries)

- Citrus fruits (oranges, lemons, grapefruits)

- Apples

- Bananas

- Kiwi

- Pineapple

- Avocado

Vegetables:

- Leafy greens (spinach, kale, Swiss chard)

- Cruciferous vegetables (broccoli, cauliflower, Brussels sprouts)

- Tomatoes

- Bell peppers

- Carrots

- Zucchini

- Mushrooms

- Onions

- Garlic

Whole Grains:

- Quinoa

- Brown rice

- Whole wheat bread

- Whole grain pasta

- Oats

Healthy Fats:

- Avocado

- Nuts (walnuts, almonds, pistachios)

- Seeds (flaxseeds, chia seeds, pumpkin seeds)

- Olive oil

- Avocado oil

Herbs and Spices:

- Turmeric

- Ginger

- Cinnamon

- Garlic powder

- Rosemary

- Thyme

- Basil

- Parsley

Dairy Alternatives:

- Almond milk

- Coconut milk

- Soy milk

Beverages:

- Water (still or sparkling)

- Green tea

- Herbal teas (peppermint, chamomile)

Miscellaneous:

- Vinegar (apple cider vinegar, balsamic vinegar)

- Low-sodium broth or stock

- Natural sweeteners (stevia, honey, maple syrup)

- Dark chocolate (in moderation, with at least 70% cocoa content)

- Nutritional yeast (for added flavor and nutrients)

When shopping for fatty liver-friendly foods, opt for fresh, whole foods whenever possible and minimize the consumption of processed and packaged foods high in unhealthy fats, sugars, and additives.

Remember to read food labels carefully and choose products with minimal added sugars, trans fats, and sodium.

Additionally, aim to incorporate a variety of colors and textures into your meals to ensure a diverse nutrient intake and promote overall health and well-being.

Foods to Avoid

For individuals with fatty liver disease, it's essential to avoid certain foods and beverages that can exacerbate liver damage, promote inflammation, and contribute to the progression of the condition. Here are foods to avoid for fatty liver:

1. Sugary Foods and Beverages:

Avoid sugary snacks, desserts, and beverages such as soda, fruit juices, energy drinks, sweetened teas, and flavored coffee drinks. These products are high in added sugars, which can contribute to liver fat accumulation and insulin resistance.

2. Processed Foods:

Limit consumption of processed and packaged foods, including fast food, chips, cookies, pastries, and other convenience snacks. These foods are often high in unhealthy fats, sugars, sodium, and additives that can contribute to liver inflammation and damage.

3. High-Fat Foods:

Avoid foods high in saturated and trans fats, such as fatty cuts of meat, fried foods, processed meats (sausage, bacon, hot dogs), butter, margarine, and hydrogenated oils. These fats can increase liver fat accumulation and promote inflammation.

4. Alcohol:

Individuals with fatty liver disease, especially alcoholic fatty liver disease (AFLD), should avoid or limit alcohol consumption. Alcohol is metabolized by the liver and can cause liver inflammation, damage, and fatty liver disease progression.

5. Simple Carbohydrates:

Limit intake of refined carbohydrates and foods made with white flour, such as white bread, white rice, pasta, and pastries. These foods can spike blood sugar levels and contribute to insulin resistance, which worsens liver health.

6. High-Sodium Foods:

Reduce consumption of high-sodium foods, including processed meats, canned soups, salty snacks, and fast food. Excess sodium intake can lead to fluid retention and worsen liver swelling and inflammation.

7. Artificial Sweeteners:

Limit the use of artificial sweeteners such as aspartame, saccharin, and sucralose. While they are low in calories, some research suggests that artificial sweeteners may disrupt gut bacteria and contribute to metabolic dysfunction.

8. Highly Processed Foods:

Avoid highly processed foods with long ingredient lists and artificial additives. Opt for whole, minimally processed foods whenever possible to support liver health and overall well-being.

By avoiding these foods and making healthier dietary choices, individuals with fatty liver disease can help reduce liver fat accumulation, inflammation, and disease progression.

It's essential to focus on a balanced diet rich in fruits, vegetables, whole grains, lean proteins, and healthy fats to support liver health and overall wellness.

CHAPTER 4

Breakfast Recipes

1. Avocado Toast with Poached Egg

Ingredients:

- 1 ripe avocado
- 2 slices of whole grain bread
- 2 eggs
- Salt and pepper to taste

Preparation:

1.   Toast the slices of whole grain bread.

2.   Mash the ripe avocado and spread it evenly on the toast.

3.   Poach the eggs to your desired level of doneness.

4. Place the poached eggs on top of the avocado toast.

5. Season with salt and pepper to make it tasty.

Nutritional Value (per serving):

- Calories: 300

- Protein: 12g

- Fat: 18g

- Carbohydrates: 25g

Cooking Time: 15 minutes

____

____

____

____

____

Progress Report:

____

____

____

____

____

2. Oatmeal with Fresh Berries

Ingredients:

- ½ cup rolled oats

- 1 cup unsweetened almond milk

- ½ cup fresh berries (such as strawberries, blueberries, or raspberries)

- 1 tablespoon honey or maple syrup (optional)

Preparation:

1. Heat the almond milk in a saucepan until it begins to gently boil.

2. Stir in the rolled oats and reduce heat to low. Cook for 5-7 minutes, stirring occasionally, until the oats are creamy.

3. Take off the heat and allow to cool a little.

4.   Top the oatmeal with fresh berries and drizzle with honey or maple syrup, if desired.

Nutritional Value (per serving):

- Calories: 250

- Protein: 6g

- Fat: 4g

- Carbohydrates: 45g

Cooking Time: 10 minutes

Notes:

____

____

____

____

____

Progress Report:

____

____

____

____

____

3. Greek Yogurt Parfait with Nuts and Honey

- ½ cup Greek yogurt

- ¼ cup of mixed nuts (like walnuts, pecans and almonds)

- 1 tablespoon honey

- ¼ cup fresh berries

Preparation:

1. Layer the Greek yogurt, mixed nuts, and fresh berries in a glass or bowl.

2. Drizzle with honey.

3. Repeat the layers if desired.

Nutritional Value (per serving):

- Calories: 300

- Protein: 15g

- Fat: 18g

- Carbohydrates: 25g

Cooking Time: 5 minutes

Notes:

____

____

____

____

____

Progress Report:

____

____

____

____

____

4. Quinoa Breakfast Bowl with Almond Milk

Ingredients:

- ½ cup cooked quinoa

- ½ cup unsweetened almond milk

- ¼ cup sliced almonds

- ¼ cup diced fruits (such as apples or berries)

- 1 tablespoon honey or maple syrup (optional)

Preparation:

1. In a bowl, combine the cooked quinoa and unsweetened almond milk.

2. Top with sliced almonds and diced fruits.

3. Drizzle with honey or maple syrup, if desired.

Nutritional Value (per serving):

- Calories: 280

- Protein: 8g

- Fat: 10g

- Carbohydrates: 40g

Cooking Time: 15 minutes

____

____

____

____

____

____

____

____

____

____

5. Vegetable Frittata with Egg Whites

Ingredients:

- 4 egg whites

- ½ cup chopped veggies (such as spinach, bell peppers, and onions)

- 1 tablespoon olive oil

- Salt and pepper to taste

Preparation:

1. Preheat the oven to 350°F (175°C).

2. A skillet with medium heat should be used to heat the olive oil.

3. Add the chopped vegetables and sauté until tender.

4. In a bowl, whisk the egg whites with salt and pepper.

5. Pour the egg whites over the sautéed vegetables in the skillet.

6. Cook for 2-3 minutes, then transfer the skillet to the oven.

7. Bake for 10-12 minutes, or until the frittata is set and lightly golden.

Nutritional Value (per serving):

- Calories: 150

- Protein: 15g

- Fat: 7g

- Carbohydrates: 8g

Cooking Time: 20 minutes

Notes:

58

____

____

____

____

____

Progress Report:

____

____

____

____

____

6. Chia Seed Pudding with Fruit Compote

Ingredients:

- 2 tablespoons chia seeds

- ½ cup unsweetened almond milk

- ½ cup mixed berries

- 1 tablespoon honey or maple syrup (optional)

Preparation:

1. In a bowl, mix the chia seeds and unsweetened almond milk. Let sit for 10 minutes, stirring occasionally, until thickened.

2. In a small saucepan, heat the mixed berries over medium heat until they release their juices and become syrupy.

3. Serve the chia seed pudding topped with the fruit compote.

4. Drizzle with honey or maple syrup, if desired.

Nutritional Value (per serving):

- Calories: 180

- Protein: 4g

- Fat: 8g

- Carbohydrates: 25g

Cooking Time: 15 minutes

Notes:

____

____

____

____

____

Progress Report:

____

____

____

____

____

7. Banana Walnut Muffins

- 1 ripe banana, mashed

- ¼ cup unsweetened applesauce

- ¼ cup almond milk

- 1 cup whole wheat flour

- ½ cup chopped walnuts

- ¼ cup honey or maple syrup

- 1 teaspoon baking powder

- ½ teaspoon cinnamon

- Pinch of salt

Preparation:

1. Preheat the oven to 350°F(175°C). Line a muffin tin with paper liners.

2. In a bowl, mix the mashed banana, unsweetened applesauce, almond milk, and honey or maple syrup.

3. In another bowl, whisk together the whole wheat flour, baking powder, cinnamon, and salt.

4. Gradually add the dry ingredients to the wet ingredients, stirring until combined.

5. Fold in the chopped walnuts.

6. Evenly distribute the batter among the muffin tins.

7. Bake for 18-20 minutes, or until a toothpick inserted into the center comes out clean.

Nutritional Value (per serving – 1 muffin):

- Calories: 150

- Protein: 4g

- Fat: 6g

- Carbohydrates: 20g

Cooking Time: 25 minutes

Notes:

____

____

____

____

____

Progress Report:

____

____

____

____

____

8. Blueberry Almond Overnight Oats

Ingredients:

- ½ cup rolled oats

- ½ cup unsweetened almond milk

- ¼ cup blueberries

- 1 tablespoon almond butter

- 1 tablespoon honey or maple syrup (optional)

Preparation:

1. In a jar or bowl, combine the rolled oats and unsweetened almond milk.

2. Stir in the blueberries and almond butter.

3. Drizzle with honey or maple syrup, if desired.

4. Cover and refrigerate overnight.

5. In the morning, stir the oats well and enjoy cold or warmed up.

Nutritional Value (per serving):

- Calories: 250

- Protein: 8g

- Fat: 10g

- Carbohydrates: 35g

Cooking Time: Overnight (no cooking required)

Notes:

____

____

____

____

____

Progress Report:

____

____

____

____

____

9. Fruit Salad with Mint and Lime Dressing

Ingredients:

- 1 cup mixed fruits (such as strawberries, kiwi, pineapple, and grapes), chopped
- 1 tablespoon fresh lime juice
- 1 tablespoon honey
- 1 tablespoon fresh mint leaves, chopped

Preparation:

1. Combine the mixed fruits in a bowl.

2. In a separate small bowl, whisk together the fresh lime juice, honey, and chopped mint leaves.

3. Drizzle the dressing over the fruit salad and toss gently to coat.

4. Serve right away or put in the fridge until you're ready to eat.

Nutritional Value (per serving):

- Calories: 80

- Protein: 1g

- Fat: 0g

- Carbohydrates: 20g

Cooking Time: 10 minutes

Notes:

____

____

____

____

____

Progress Report:

____

____

____

____

____

10. Veggie and Mushroom Scramble

Ingredients:

- 2 eggs

- ¼ cup sliced mushrooms

- ¼ cup chopped bell peppers

- ¼ cup chopped onions

- 1 tablespoon olive oil

- Salt and pepper to taste

Preparation:

1. In a bowl, whisk the eggs until well beaten. Set aside.

2. Heat olive oil in a skillet over medium heat.

3. Add the chopped onions and cook until translucent.

4. Add the sliced mushrooms and bell peppers to the skillet. Cook until vegetables are tender.

5. Transfer the whisked eggs into the frying pan.

6. Gently scramble the eggs with the vegetables until cooked through.

7. Season with salt and pepper to make it tasty.

Nutritional Value (per serving):

- Calories: 180

- Protein: 10g

- Fat: 12g

- Carbohydrates: 5g

Cooking Time: 10 minutes

Notes:

____

____

____

____

____

Progress Report:

____

____

____

____

____

CHAPTER 5

Lunch Recipes

1. Baked Salmon with Steamed Asparagus

Ingredients:

- 2 salmon fillets
- 1 bunch asparagus
- Olive oil
- Salt and pepper to taste

Preparation:

1. Set the oven to 375°F (190°C) heat

2. Ensure the salmon fillets is put on a baking pan covered with parchment paper.

3. Drizzle salmon with olive oil and season with salt and pepper.

4. Arrange asparagus around the salmon.

5. Bake for 12-15 minutes or until salmon is cooked through and asparagus is tender.

Nutritional Value:

- Calories: 300 kcal

- Protein: 30g

- Fat: 15g

- Carbohydrates: 5g

Cooking Time: 15 minutes

Notes:

____

____

____

____

____

Progress Report:

____

____

____

____

____

2. Stuffed Bell Peppers with Quinoa and Lentils

- 4 bell peppers

- 1 cup cooked quinoa

- 1 cup cooked lentils

- ½ cup diced tomatoes

- ¼ cup chopped onion

- ¼ cup chopped parsley

- Salt and pepper to taste

1. Set the oven to 375°F (190°C) heat

2. Removed tops and seeds of the bell peppers

3. In a bowl, mix cooked quinoa, cooked lentils, diced tomatoes, chopped onion, chopped parsley, salt, and pepper.

4. Stuff the bell peppers with the quinoa-lentil mixture.

5. Place the stuffed peppers in a baking dish and cover with foil.

6. Bake for 25-30 minutes or until peppers are tender.

Nutritional Value:

- Calories: 250 kcal

- Protein: 12g

- Fat: 2g

- Carbohydrates: 45g

Cooking Time: 30 minutes

Notes:

____

____

____

____

____

Progress Report:

____

____

____

____

____

3. Chickpea and Roasted Vegetable Bowl

Ingredients:

- 1 can of chickpeas, that is drained and rinsed
- 2 cups mixed roasted vegetables (bell peppers, zucchini, eggplant)
- 1 cup cooked quinoa
- ¼ cup crumbled feta cheese
- 2 tablespoons chopped fresh parsley
- Lemon vinaigrette dressing

Preparation:

1. In a bowl, combine chickpeas, roasted vegetables, cooked quinoa, crumbled feta cheese, and chopped parsley.

2. Add a lemon vinaigrette dressing drizzle and toss to coat.

Nutritional Value:

- Calories: 350 kcal

- Protein: 15g

- Fat: 8g

- Carbohydrates: 55g

Cooking Time: 25 minutes

Notes:

____

____

____

____

____

Progress Report:

____

____

____

____

____

4. Brown Rice and Grilled Chicken Bowl

Ingredients:

- 1 cup cooked brown rice

- 4 oz grilled chicken breast, sliced

- 1 cup steamed broccoli florets

- ¼ cup sliced carrots

- 2 tablespoons soy sauce

- 1 tablespoon sesame seeds

Preparation:

1. Divide cooked brown rice, grilled chicken breast slices, steamed broccoli florets, and sliced carrots among serving bowls.

2. Drizzle with soy sauce and sprinkle with sesame seeds.

Nutritional Value:

- Calories: 400 kcal

- Protein: 30g

- Fat: 8g

- Carbohydrates: 55g

Cooking Time: 20 minutes

____

____

____

____

____

____

____

____

____

____

5. Quinoa and Black Bean Salad

Ingredients:

- 1 cup cooked quinoa

- 1 can drained black beans, and rinsed

- 1 cup cherry tomatoes, halved

- ¼ cup diced red onion

- ¼ cup chopped cilantro

- Juice of 1 lime

- 2 tablespoons olive oil

- Salt and pepper to taste

Preparation:

1. In a large bowl, combine cooked quinoa, black beans, cherry tomatoes, diced red onion, and chopped cilantro.

2. Ensure you drizzle with lime juice and olive oil.

3. Season with salt and pepper to taste and toss to combine.

Nutritional Value:

- Calories: 300 kcal

- Protein: 12g

- Fat: 8g

- Carbohydrates: 45g

Cooking Time: 15 minutes

Notes:

____

____

____

____

____

Progress Report:

____

____

____

____

____

6. Sauteed Spinach and Mushroom Quesadilla

Ingredients:

- 2 whole grain tortillas

- 1 cup spinach leaves

- ½ cup sliced mushrooms

- ¼ cup shredded mozzarella cheese

- ¼ cup diced tomatoes

- ¼ cup diced onion

- 1 clove garlic, minced

- Olive oil for sautéing

- Salt and pepper to taste

Preparation:

1. In a skillet, heat olive oil over medium heat. Add minced garlic and diced onion, sauté until softened.

2. Add sliced mushrooms and cook until they release their moisture.

3. Cook the spinach until the leaves have wilted. Season with salt and pepper.

4. Place one tortilla in the skillet, sprinkle with shredded mozzarella cheese, and top with the sautéed spinach and mushroom mixture and diced tomatoes.

5. Gently press down on the second tortilla after placing it on top.

6. Cook until the bottom tortilla is crispy and the cheese is melted, then flip and cook the other side.

Nutritional Value:

- Calories: 300 kcal

- Protein: 12g

- Fat: 10g

- Carbohydrates: 40g

Cooking Time: 15 minutes

Notes:

____

____

____

____

____

Progress Report:

____

____

____

____

____

7. Tofu Stir Fry with Colorful Veggies

- 1 block of firm tofu, that is pressed and cubed

- 2 cups mixed colorful veggies (like bell peppers, broccoli, carrots, snap peas)

- 2 tablespoons soy sauce

- 1 tablespoon sesame oil

- 1 tablespoon rice vinegar

- 1 teaspoon minced ginger

- 1 clove garlic, minced

- Salt and pepper to taste

- Cooked brown rice for serving

Preparation:

1. In a skillet, heat sesame oil over medium heat. Add the ginger and garlic, minced, and sauté until fragrant.

2. Add cubed tofu to the skillet and cook until golden brown on all sides.

3. Add mixed colorful vegetables to the skillet and stir-fry until tender-crisp.

4. In a small bowl, mix soy sauce and rice vinegar, then pour over the tofu and vegetables.

5. Stir well to coat everything evenly. Season with salt and pepper to make it tasty.

6. Serve over cooked brown rice.

Nutritional Value:

- Calories: 350 kcal

- Protein: 20g

- Fat: 15g

- Carbohydrates: 30g

Notes:

____

____

____

____

____

Progress Report:

____

____

____

____

____

8. Eggplant and Chickpea Curry

Ingredients:

- 1 large eggplant, diced

- 1 can of chickpeas, that is drained and rinsed

- 1 onion, diced

- 2 cloves garlic, minced

- 1 tablespoon curry powder

- 1 teaspoon ground cumin

- 1 teaspoon ground coriander

- 1 can diced tomatoes

- 1 cup vegetable broth

- 2 tablespoons chopped fresh cilantro

- Salt and pepper to taste

- Cooked brown rice for serving

1. In a large pot, heat olive oil over medium heat. Add diced onion and minced garlic, sauté until softened.

2. Add diced eggplant to the pot and cook until slightly browned.

3. Stir in curry powder, ground cumin, and ground coriander, and cook for another minute.

4. Add diced tomatoes, chickpeas, and vegetable broth to the pot. Bring to a simmer and cook for 15-20 minutes until the eggplant is tender.

5. Season with salt and pepper to taste, and garnish with chopped fresh cilantro.

6. Serve over cooked brown rice.

Nutritional Value:

- Calories: 320 kcal

- Protein: 12g

- Fat: 8g

- Carbohydrates: 50g

Cooking Time: 30 minutes

Notes:

____

____

____

____

____

Progress Report:

____

____

____

____

____

9. Baked Cod with Lemon and Herb

Ingredients:

- 2 cod fillets

- 2 tablespoons olive oil

- 2 cloves garlic, minced

- 1 tablespoon lemon juice

- 1 teaspoon lemon zest

- 1 teaspoon dried thyme

- Salt and pepper to taste

Preparation:

1. Set the oven to 375°F (190°C) heat.

2. Place cod fillets in a baking dish lined with parchment paper.

3. In a small bowl, whisk together olive oil, minced garlic, lemon juice, lemon zest, dried thyme, salt, and pepper.

4. Pour the mixture over the cod fillets, ensuring they are evenly coated.

5. Bake for 15-20 minutes or until the fish is opaque and flakes easily with a fork.

Nutritional Value:

- Calories: 200 kcal

- Protein: 25g

- Fat: 8g

- Carbohydrates: 2g

Cooking Time: 20 minutes

Notes:

____

____

____

____

____

Progress Report:

____

____

____

____

____

10. Sweet Potato and Black Bean Chili

Ingredients:

- 2 sweet potatoes, diced
- 1 can of drained black beans, and rinsed
- 1 can diced tomatoes
- 1 onion, diced
- 2 cloves garlic, minced
- 1 tablespoon chili powder
- 1 teaspoon ground cumin
- ½ teaspoon smoked paprika
- 2 cups vegetable broth
- Salt and pepper to taste

1. In a large pot, heat olive oil over medium heat. Add diced onion and minced garlic, sauté until softened.

2. Add diced sweet potatoes to the pot and cook until slightly softened.

3. Stir in chili powder, ground cumin, and smoked paprika, and cook for another minute.

4. Add black beans, diced tomatoes, and vegetable broth to the pot. Bring to a simmer and cook for 20-25 minutes until sweet potatoes are tender.

5. Season with salt and pepper to make it tasty.

6. Serve hot, garnished with chopped fresh cilantro or green onions if desired.

Nutritional Value:

- Calories: 250 kcal

- Protein: 10g

- Fat: 1g

- Carbohydrates: 50g

Cooking Time: 30 minutes

Notes:

____

____

____

____

____

Progress Report:

____

____

____

____

____

CHAPTER 6

Dinner Recipes

1. Baked Chicken Meatloaf with Spinach

Ingredients:

- 1 lb ground chicken

- 1 cup chopped spinach

- ¼ cup breadcrumbs

- 1 egg

- ¼ cup grated Parmesan cheese

- 1 teaspoon garlic powder

- Salt and pepper to taste

1. Preheat oven to 375°F (190°C).

2. In a bowl, combine ground chicken, chopped spinach, breadcrumbs, egg, Parmesan cheese, garlic powder, salt, and pepper.

3. Mix until well combined, then shape into a loaf and place in a baking dish.

4. Bake for 40-45 minutes or until cooked through.

Nutritional Value (per serving):

- Calories: 250 kcal

- Protein: 25g

- Fat: 10g

- Carbohydrates: 15g

Cooking Time: 45 minutes

Notes:

____

____

____

____

____

Progress Report:

____

____

____

____

____

2. Pork Stir Fry with Bok Choy and Garlic

- 1 lb of pork loin, that is thinly sliced

- 2 cups bok choy, chopped

- 3 cloves garlic, minced

- 2 tablespoons soy sauce

- 1 tablespoon oyster sauce

- 1 tablespoon sesame oil

- 1 tablespoon olive oil

- Salt and pepper to taste

Preparation:

1. A skillet with medium heat should be used to heat the olive oil. Add the garlic minced, and sauté until fragrant.

2. Add thinly sliced pork loin and stir-fry until browned.

3. Add chopped bok choy and continue to stir-fry until tender.

4. Stir in soy sauce, oyster sauce, and sesame oil. Season with salt and pepper to make it tasty.

5. Cook for an additional 2-3 minutes, then serve hot.

Nutritional Value (per serving):

- Calories: 300 kcal

- Protein: 25g

- Fat: 15g

- Carbohydrates: 10g

Cooking Time: 20 minutes

Notes:

____

____

____

____

____

Progress Report:

____

____

____

____

____

3. Turkey and Vegetable Stir Fry

Ingredients:

- 1 lb ground turkey

- 2 cups mixed vegetables (bell peppers, broccoli, carrots)

- 2 cloves garlic, minced

- 2 tablespoons soy sauce

- 1 tablespoon olive oil

- 1 teaspoon sesame oil

- Salt and pepper to taste

Preparation:

1. A skillet with medium heat should be used to heat the olive oil.Add minced garlic and cook until fragrant.

2. Add ground turkey and cook until browned.

3. Add mixed vegetables and stir-fry until tender-crisp.

4. Add sesame oil and soy sauce and stir. Season with salt and pepper to make it tasty.

5. Cook for an additional 2-3 minutes, then serve hot.

Nutritional Value (per serving):

- Calories: 280 kcal

- Protein: 20g

- Fat: 10g

- Carbohydrates: 15g

Cooking Time: 20 minutes

Notes:

____

____

____

____

____

Progress Report:

____

____

____

____

____

4. Baked Salmon with Dijon Mustard Glaze

Ingredients:

- 4 salmon fillets

- 2 tablespoons Dijon mustard

- 1 tablespoon honey

- 1 tablespoon olive oil

- 1 teaspoon minced garlic

- Salt and pepper to taste

Preparation:

1. Set the oven to 375°F (190°C) heat.

2. In a small bowl, mix together Dijon mustard, honey, olive oil, minced garlic, salt, and pepper.

3. Ensure the salmon fillets is put on a baking pan covered with parchment paper.

4. Brush the mustard glaze over the salmon fillets.

5. Bake the salmon for 12 to 15 minutes, or until it is cooked through and flake readily when tested with a fork.

Nutritional Value (per serving):

- Calories: 300 kcal
- Protein: 25g
- Fat: 15g
- Carbohydrates: 8g

Cooking Time: 15 minutes

____

____

____

____

____

Progress Report:

____

____

____

____

____

5. Herb-Marinated Grilled Pork Chops

Ingredients:

- 4 pork chops

- 2 tablespoons olive oil

- 2 cloves garlic, minced

- 1 tablespoon of chopped fresh herbs (like thyme, sage or rosemary)

- Salt and pepper to taste

Preparation:

1. In a small bowl, combine olive oil, minced garlic, chopped herbs, salt, and pepper.

2. Place pork chops in a shallow dish and pour the marinade over them, turning to coat.

3. Cover and refrigerate for at least 30 minutes, or overnight for best flavor.

4. Preheat grill to medium-high heat. Remove pork chops from marinade and discard excess marinade.

5. Grill pork chops for 5-6 minutes per side, or until cooked through.

Nutritional Value (per serving):
- Calories: 280 kcal
- Protein: 30g
- Fat: 15g
- Carbohydrates: 2g

Cooking Time: 12 minutes

Notes:

____

____

____

____

____

Progress Report:

____

____

____

____

____

6. Lean Beef and Vegetable Stir Fry

Ingredients:

- 1 lb lean beef (such as sirloin or flank steak), thinly sliced

- 2 cups mixed veggies (like bell peppers, broccoli, snap peas)

- 2 cloves garlic, minced

- 2 tablespoons soy sauce

- 1 tablespoon hoisin sauce

- 1 tablespoon olive oil

- Salt and pepper to taste

1. A skillet with high heat should be used to heat the olive oil. Add garlic, minced and sauté until fragrant.

2. Add thinly sliced beef and stir-fry until browned.

3. Add mixed vegetables and continue to stir-fry until tender-crisp.

4. Stir in soy sauce and hoisin sauce. Season with salt and pepper to make it tasty.

5. Cook for an additional 2-3 minutes, then serve hot.

Nutritional Value (per serving):

- Calories: 280 kcal

- Protein: 25g

- Fat: 12g

- Carbohydrates: 15g

Cooking Time: 15 minutes

Notes:

____

____

____

____

____

Progress Report:

____

____

____

____

____

7. Baked Cod with Lentil Dill

- 4 cod fillets

- 1 cup cooked lentils

- 2 tablespoons chopped fresh dill

- 1 lemon, juiced and zested

- 2 cloves garlic, minced

- 2 tablespoons olive oil

- Salt and pepper to taste

Preparation:

1. Set the oven to 375°F (190°C) heat.

2. In a bowl, combine cooked lentils, chopped fresh dill, minced garlic, lemon juice, lemon zest, olive oil, salt, and pepper.

3. Ensure you place cod fillets on a baking sheet lined with parchment paper.

4. Spoon the lentil mixture over the cod fillets.

5. Bake for 15-20 minutes, or until the cod is cooked through and flakes easily with a fork.

Nutritional Value (per serving):

- Calories: 250 kcal

- Protein: 25g

- Fat: 10g

- Carbohydrates: 15g

Cooking Time: 20 minutes

Notes:

____

____

____

____

____

Progress Report:

____

____

____

____

____

8. Steamed Fish with Ginger and Soy Sauce

Ingredients:

- 4 white fish fillets (such as tilapia or halibut)
- 2 tablespoons soy sauce
- 1 tablespoon rice vinegar
- 1 tablespoon sesame oil
- 1 tablespoon minced fresh ginger
- 2 cloves garlic, minced
- 2 green onions, thinly sliced

Preparation:

1. In a shallow dish, mix together soy sauce, rice vinegar, sesame oil, minced ginger, minced garlic, and sliced green onions.

2. Place fish fillets in a steamer basket and set over a pot of boiling water.

3. Brush the fish fillets with the soy sauce mixture.

4. Cover and steam for 8-10 minutes, or until the fish is cooked through and flakes easily with a fork.

Nutritional Value (per serving):

- Calories: 200 kcal
- Protein: 25g
- Fat: 8g
- Carbohydrates: 5g

Cooking Time: 10 minutes

Notes:

____

____

____

____

____

Progress Report:

____

____

____

____

____

9. Grilled Skinless Chicken Breast with Herbs

Ingredients:

- 4 skinless chicken breast fillets

- 2 tablespoons olive oil

- 2 cloves garlic, minced

- 1 tablespoon chopped fresh herbs (such as rosemary, thyme, or oregano)

- Salt and pepper to taste

Preparation:

1. Preheat grill to medium-high heat.

2. In a small bowl, mix together olive oil, minced garlic, chopped fresh herbs, salt, and pepper.

3. Brush the herb mixture over the chicken breast fillets.

4. Grill chicken breast fillets for 6-7 minutes per side, or until cooked through and no longer pink in the center.

Nutritional Value (per serving):
- Calories: 220 kcal
- Protein: 30g
- Fat: 10g
- Carbohydrates: 1g

Cooking Time: 15 minutes

____

____

____

____

____

Progress Report:

____

____

____

____

10. Beef Stir Fry with Broccoli and Snow Peas

Ingredients:

- 1 lb beef sirloin, thinly sliced
- 2 cups broccoli florets
- 1 cup snow peas, trimmed
- 1 red bell pepper, sliced
- 2 cloves garlic, minced
- 2 tablespoons soy sauce
- 1 tablespoon oyster sauce
- 1 tablespoon sesame oil
- 1 tablespoon cornstarch
- Salt and pepper to taste
- Cooked rice, for serving

1. In a bowl, whisk together soy sauce, oyster sauce, sesame oil, cornstarch, salt, and pepper. Set aside.

2. In a large skillet or wok, heat up one tablespoon of oil over high heat. Add minced garlic and stir-fry for 30 seconds.

3. Add beef slices and stir-fry until browned. Remove from skillet and set aside.

4. In the same skillet, add a little more oil if needed. Add broccoli florets, snow peas, and sliced red bell pepper. When the vegetables are crisp-tender, stir-fry them for 3–4 minutes.

5. Return the cooked beef to the skillet. Pour the sauce over the beef and vegetables, stirring until everything is well coated and the sauce has thickened.

6. Serve hot over cooked rice.

Nutritional Value (per serving, without rice):

- Calories: 280 kcal

- Protein: 25g

- Fat: 12g

- Carbohydrates: 15g

Cooking Time: 20 minutes

Notes:

____

____

____

____

____

Progress Report:

____

____

____

____

____

CHAPTER 7

Snack Recipes

1. Roasted Radishes

Ingredients:

- 1 bunch radishes, trimmed and halved

- 1 tablespoon olive oil

- Salt and pepper to taste

Preparation:

1. Preheat the oven to 400°F (200°C).

2. Toss radishes with olive oil, salt, and pepper.

3. Spread radishes on a baking sheet lined with parchment paper.

4. Roast for 15-20 minutes, or until radishes are tender and slightly caramelized.

- Calories: 40 kcal

- Protein: 1g

- Fat: 3g

- Carbohydrates: 3g

Cooking Time: 20 minutes

____

____

____

____

____

Progress Report:

____

____

____

____

____

2. Mango and Watermelon Salsa

Ingredients:

- 1 cup diced mango

- 1 cup diced watermelon

- ¼ cup finely chopped red onion

- 1 jalapeno, seeded and finely chopped

- ¼ cup chopped fresh cilantro

- Juice of 1 lime

- Salt to taste

Preparation:

1. In a bowl, combine diced mango, diced watermelon, chopped red onion, chopped jalapeno, chopped cilantro, lime juice, and salt.

2. Mix well until evenly combined.

3. Serve chilled as a dip or topping for grilled meats or fish.

Nutritional Value (per serving):

- Calories: 45 kcal

- Protein: 1g

- Fat: 0g

- Carbohydrates: 11g

Preparation Time: 10 minutes

Notes:

____

____

____

____

____

Progress Report:

____

____

____

____

____

3. Spiced French Toast

- 4 slices whole grain bread

- 2 eggs

- ¼ cup milk (or almond milk)

- 1 teaspoon ground cinnamon

- ½ teaspoon vanilla extract

- 1 tablespoon olive oil

Preparation:

1. Whisk the eggs, milk, ground cinnamon, and vanilla extract in a shallow dish.

 2. Dip each slice of bread into the egg mixture, coating both sides evenly.

3. Heat olive oil in a non-stick skillet over medium heat.

4. Cook each slice of bread for 2-3 minutes on each side, or until golden brown and cooked through.

Nutritional Value (per serving):

- Calories: 150 kcal

- Protein: 8g

- Fat: 6g

- Carbohydrates: 18g

Cooking Time: 10 minutes per batch (2 slices)

4. Radish Hash Browns

Ingredients:

- 2 cups grated radishes

- 1 egg

- 2 tablespoons almond flour

- ¼ teaspoon garlic powder

- Salt and pepper to taste

- 2 tablespoons olive oil

Preparation:

1. Place grated radishes in a clean kitchen towel and squeeze out excess moisture.

2. In a bowl, combine grated radishes, egg, almond flour, garlic powder, salt, and pepper. Mix well.

3. In a skillet over medium heat, heat the olive oil.

4. Form radish mixture into small patties and place them in the skillet.

5. Cook for 4-5 minutes on each side, or until golden brown and crispy.

Nutritional Value (per serving):

- Calories: 90 kcal

- Protein: 3g

- Fat: 7g

- Carbohydrates: 5g

Cooking Time: 10 minutes

Notes:

____

____

____

____

____

Progress Report:

____

____

____

____

____

5. Chilled Mango Treat

Ingredients:

- 1 ripe mango, peeled and diced
- ½ cup plain Greek yogurt
- 1 tablespoon honey (optional)
- Fresh mint leaves for garnish

Preparation:

1. Place diced mango in a blender or food processor and puree until smooth.

2. In a bowl, mix together mango puree, Greek yogurt, and honey (if using).

3. Transfer the mixture to individual serving cups or bowls.

4. Chill in the refrigerator for at least 1 hour before serving.

5. Garnish with fresh mint leaves before serving.

Nutritional Value (per serving):

- Calories: 100 kcal

- Protein: 5g

- Fat: 1g

- Carbohydrates: 20g

Preparation Time: 5 minutes

Progress Report:

6. Walnut and Spiced Apple Tonic

- 1 apple, sliced

- 1 tablespoon chopped walnuts

- ½ teaspoon ground cinnamon

- Pinch of ground nutmeg

- Pinch of ground cloves

- 1 cup water

- Ice cubes

1. In a saucepan, combine apple slices, chopped walnuts, ground cinnamon, nutmeg, cloves, and water.

2. Bring to a boil, then reduce heat and simmer for 5-7 minutes.

3. Take off from the heat and allow to cool slightly.

4. Strain the mixture and discard the solids.

5. Serve the spiced apple tonic over ice cubes.

Nutritional Value (per serving):

- Calories: 50 kcal

- Protein: 1g

- Fat: 2g

- Carbohydrates: 10g

Cooking Time: 10 minutes

Notes:

___

___

___

___

___

Progress Report:

___

___

___

___

___

7. Spiced Apricot Sesame Balls

- 1 cup dried apricots

- ½ cup rolled oats

- ¼ cup sesame seeds

- ¼ cup unsweetened shredded coconut

- ½ teaspoon ground cinnamon

- ¼ teaspoon ground ginger

- 2 tablespoons honey

- Water (as needed)

Preparation:

1. Place dried apricots in a food processor and pulse until finely chopped.

2. Add rolled oats, sesame seeds, shredded coconut, ground cinnamon, ground ginger, and honey to the food processor.

3. Process until the mixture comes together. If the mixture is too dry, add water, a tablespoon at a time, until it reaches a sticky consistency.

4. Roll the mixture into small balls using your hands.

5. Before serving, place the balls on a parchment paper-lined baking sheet and chill for at least half an hour.

Nutritional Value (per serving, about 2 balls):

- Calories: 100 kcal
- Protein: 2g
- Fat: 4g
- Carbohydrates: 16g

Preparation Time: 15 minutes

Notes:

____

____

____

____

____

Progress Report:

____

____

____

____

____

8. Grape Celery and Parsley Reviver

- 1 cup seedless grapes
- 2 celery stalks
- ¼ cup fresh parsley leaves
- 1 cup water
- Ice cubes

1. Wash grapes, celery stalks, and parsley leaves under cold water.

2. Trim the ends of the celery stalks and cut them into smaller pieces.

3. In a blender, combine grapes, celery pieces, parsley leaves, and water.

4. Blend until smooth.

5. Pour the mixture into glasses filled with ice cubes.

Nutritional Value (per serving):

- Calories: 60 kcal

- Protein: 1g

- Fat: 0g

- Carbohydrates: 15g

Preparation Time: 5 minutes

Notes:

____

____

____

____

____

Progress Report:

____

____

____

____

____

9. Tuna Salad

Ingredients:

- 1 can of tuna in water, and drained
- ¼ cup diced cucumber
- ¼ cup diced red bell pepper
- 1 tablespoon chopped fresh parsley
- 1 tablespoon olive oil
- 1 tablespoon lemon juice
- Salt and pepper to taste

Preparation:

1. In a bowl, combine drained tuna, diced cucumber, diced red bell pepper, chopped parsley, olive oil, lemon juice, salt, and pepper.

2. Mix well until everything is evenly combined.

3. Serve chilled as a salad or on whole grain bread as a sandwich filling.

Nutritional Value (per serving):

- Calories: 150 kcal

- Protein: 15g

- Fat: 8g

- Carbohydrates: 5g

Preparation Time: 10 minutes

Notes:

____

____

____

____

____

Progress Report:

____

____

____

____

____

10. Wheat Crackers

Ingredients:

- 1 cup whole wheat flour

- ¼ teaspoon salt

- ¼ teaspoon baking powder

- 2 tablespoons olive oil

- ¼ cup water

Preparation:

1. Set the oven to 350°F (175°C) heat and ensure to line a baking sheet with parchment paper.

2. In a bowl, combine whole wheat flour, salt, and baking powder.

3. Add olive oil and water to the dry ingredients and mix until a dough forms.

4. Roll out the dough on a lightly floured surface to about 1/8 inch thickness.

5. Use a knife or pizza cutter to cut the dough into small squares or rectangles.

6. Transfer the crackers to the prepared baking sheet and bake for 10-12 minutes, or until golden brown and crispy.

7. Let the crackers cool completely before serving.

Nutritional Value (per serving, about 6 crackers):

- Calories: 70 kcal

- Protein: 2g

- Fat: 3g

- Carbohydrates: 9g

Cooking Time: 12 minutes

Notes:

Progress Report:

30 Day Meal Plan

Week 1

Day 1:

Breakfast: Avocado Toast with Poached Egg

Lunch: Stuffed Bell Peppers with Quinoa and Lentils

Dinner: Baked Chicken Meatloaf with Spinach

Snack: Roasted Radishes

Day 2:

Breakfast: Oatmeal with Fresh Berries

Lunch: Chickpea and Roasted Vegetable Bowl

Dinner: Pork Stir Fry with Bok Choy and Garlic

Snack: Mango and Watermelon Salsa

Day 3:

Breakfast: Greek Yogurt Parfait with Nuts and Honey

Lunch: Brown Rice and Grilled Chicken Bowl

Dinner: Turkey and Vegetable Stir Fry

Snack: Spiced French Toast

Day 4:

Breakfast: Quinoa Breakfast Bowl with Almond Milk

Lunch: Quinoa and Black Bean Salad

Dinner: Baked Salmon with Dijon Mustard Glaze

Snack: Radish Hash Browns

Day 5:

Breakfast: Vegetable Frittata with Egg Whites

Lunch: Sauteed Spinach and Mushroom Quesadilla

Dinner: Herb-Marinated Grilled Pork Chops

Snack: Chilled Mango Treat

Day 6:

Breakfast: Chia Seed Pudding with Fruit Compote

Lunch: Tofu Stir Fry with Colorful Veggies

Dinner: Lean Beef and Vegetable Stir Fry

Snack: Walnut and Spiced Apple Tonic

Day 7:

Breakfast: Banana Walnut Muffins

Lunch: Eggplant and Chickpea Curry

Dinner: Baked Cod with Lentil Dill

Snack: Spiced Apricot Sesame Balls

Week 2

Breakfast: Blueberry Almond Overnight Oats

Lunch: Baked Cod with Lemon and Herb

Dinner: Steamed Fish with Ginger and Soy Sauce

Snack: Grape Celery and Parsley Reviver

Breakfast: Fruit Salad with Mint and Lime Dressing

Lunch: Sweet Potato and Black Bean Chili

Dinner: Grilled Skinless Chicken Breast with Herbs

Snack: Tuna Salad

Breakfast: Veggie and Mushroom Scramble

Lunch: Beef Stir Fry with Broccoli and Snow Peas

Dinner: Baked Chicken Meatloaf with Spinach

Snack: Wheat Crackers

Day 11:

Breakfast: Chia Seed Pudding with Fruit Compote

Lunch: Tofu Stir Fry with Colorful Veggies

Dinner: Lean Beef and Vegetable Stir Fry

Snack: Walnut and Spiced Apple Tonic

Day 12:

Breakfast: Banana Walnut Muffins

Lunch: Eggplant and Chickpea Curry

Dinner: Baked Cod with Lentil Dill

Snack: Spiced Apricot Sesame Balls

Breakfast: Blueberry Almond Overnight Oats

Lunch: Baked Cod with Lemon and Herb

Dinner: Steamed Fish with Ginger and Soy Sauce

Snack: Grape Celery and Parsley Reviver

Breakfast: Fruit Salad with Mint and Lime Dressing

Lunch: Sweet Potato and Black Bean Chili

Dinner: Grilled Skinless Chicken Breast with Herbs

Snack: Tuna Salad

Week 3

Day 15:

Breakfast: Veggie and Mushroom Scramble

Lunch: Beef Stir Fry with Broccoli and Snow Peas

Dinner: Baked Chicken Meatloaf with Spinach

Snack: Wheat Crackers

Day 16:

Breakfast: Avocado Toast with Poached Egg

Lunch: Stuffed Bell Peppers with Quinoa and Lentils

Dinner: Baked Chicken Meatloaf with Spinach

Snack: Roasted Radishes

Day 17:

Breakfast: Oatmeal with Fresh Berries

Lunch: Chickpea and Roasted Vegetable Bowl

Dinner: Pork Stir Fry with Bok Choy and Garlic

Snack: Mango and Watermelon Salsa

Day 18:

Breakfast: Greek Yogurt Parfait with Nuts and Honey

Lunch: Brown Rice and Grilled Chicken Bowl

Dinner: Turkey and Vegetable Stir Fry

Snack: Spiced French Toast

Day 19:

Breakfast: Quinoa Breakfast Bowl with Almond Milk

Lunch: Quinoa and Black Bean Salad

Dinner: Baked Salmon with Dijon Mustard Glaze

Snack: Radish Hash Browns

Day 20:

Breakfast: Vegetable Frittata with Egg Whites

Lunch: Sauteed Spinach and Mushroom Quesadilla

Dinner: Herb-Marinated Grilled Pork Chops

Snack: Chilled Mango Treat

Day 21:

Breakfast: Avocado Toast with Poached Egg

Lunch: Stuffed Bell Peppers with Quinoa and Lentils

Dinner: Baked Chicken Meatloaf with Spinach

Snack: Roasted Radishes

Week 4

Day 22:

Breakfast: Oatmeal with Fresh Berries

Lunch: Chickpea and Roasted Vegetable Bowl

Dinner: Pork Stir Fry with Bok Choy and Garlic

Snack: Mango and Watermelon Salsa

Day 23:

Breakfast: Greek Yogurt Parfait with Nuts and Honey

Lunch: Brown Rice and Grilled Chicken Bowl

Dinner: Turkey and Vegetable Stir Fry

Snack: Spiced French Toast

Day 24:

Breakfast: Quinoa Breakfast Bowl with Almond Milk

Lunch: Quinoa and Black Bean Salad

Dinner: Baked Salmon with Dijon Mustard Glaze

Snack: Radish Hash Browns

Day 25:

Breakfast: Vegetable Frittata with Egg Whites

Lunch: Sauteed Spinach and Mushroom Quesadilla

Dinner: Herb-Marinated Grilled Pork Chops

Snack: Chilled Mango Treat

Day 26:

Breakfast: Chia Seed Pudding with Fruit Compote

Lunch: Tofu Stir Fry with Colorful Veggies

Dinner: Lean Beef and Vegetable Stir Fry

Snack: Walnut and Spiced Apple Tonic

Day 27:

Breakfast: Banana Walnut Muffins

Lunch: Eggplant and Chickpea Curry

Dinner: Baked Cod with Lentil Dill

Snack: Spiced Apricot Sesame Balls

Day 28:

Breakfast: Blueberry Almond Overnight Oats

Lunch: Baked Cod with Lemon and Herb

Dinner: Steamed Fish with Ginger and Soy Sauce

Snack: Grape Celery and Parsley Reviver

Day 29:

Breakfast: Fruit Salad with Mint and Lime Dressing

Lunch: Sweet Potato and Black Bean Chili

Dinner: Grilled Skinless Chicken Breast with Herbs

Snack: Tuna Salad

Breakfast: Veggie and Mushroom Scramble

Lunch: Beef Stir Fry with Broccoli and Snow Peas

Dinner: Baked Chicken Meatloaf with Spinach

Snack: Wheat Crackers

CONCLUSION

In concluding this Fatty Liver Diet Cookbook For Seniors, I extend my heartfelt gratitude to you who have embarked on this journey towards better health. Your dedication to learning about and treating fatty liver disease is admirable, and I hope this cookbook helps you on your path to better health.

I want to sincerely wish you continued success on this path as we come to the end of this chapter. I hope every recipe in this book gives you energy and joy in your everyday life, while also providing nourishment for your body and spirit. Recall that each step you take to improve your eating habits is one step closer to taking back control of your health and raising your standard of living.

Remember that you are not alone, even though the path ahead may be difficult. You possess the ability to conquer challenges and accomplish your health objectives with commitment, endurance, and the help of this cookbook. Seize the chance presented by each meal to fuel your body, achieve internal healing, and prosper in all facets of your life.

May this cookbook be your trusted companion and guide, leading you towards lasting wellness and vitality.

Thank you for allowing me to contribute to your health journey. Here's to a healthier, happier you!

BONUS: WEIGHT LOSS EXERCISES FOR SENIORS

In addition to adopting a healthy diet, incorporating regular physical activity into your routine is essential for supporting weight loss and overall well-being. Here are some low-impact exercises tailored specifically for seniors to complement your Fatty Liver Diet journey:

1.   **Walking:** Walking is one of the simplest and most effective forms of exercise. Aim for at least 30 minutes of brisk walking each day to improve cardiovascular health and burn calories.

2.   **Water Aerobics:** Water aerobics is a gentle yet effective way to exercise without putting strain on your joints. Join a local water

aerobics class or perform simple exercises in the pool to improve strength, flexibility, and endurance.

3.   **Tai Chi:** Tai Chi is a gentle form of martial arts that focuses on slow, flowing movements and deep breathing. Practicing Tai Chi can improve balance, flexibility, and overall fitness.

4.   **Chair Yoga:** Traditional yoga poses are modified in chair yoga so that they can be done sitting down or with the assistance of a chair. It helps improve flexibility, strength, and relaxation.

5.   **Resistance Band Exercises:** Resistance bands are lightweight and portable, making them ideal for seniors. Perform exercises such as bicep curls, shoulder presses, and leg extensions to build muscle and tone your body.

6.   **Cycling:** Cycling, whether outdoors or on a stationary bike, is an excellent low-impact exercise that strengthens your legs and improves cardiovascular health.

7.   **Dancing:** Put on your favorite music and dance around your living room! Dancing is a fun way to get your heart rate up, improve coordination, and burn calories.

Remember to consult with your healthcare provider before starting any new exercise program, especially if you have existing health conditions. Begin cautiously, pay attention to your body, and progressively increase the length and intensity of your workouts. With consistency and dedication, you'll not only support your weight loss goals but also enhance your overall health and vitality.

My Little Request

Dear Reader,

Thanks for your purchase, hope you enjoyed reading.

Could you please take a few seconds to leave a positive feedback on this book?

It'll help reach more people and we can collectively reverse this deadly disease.

Thank you.

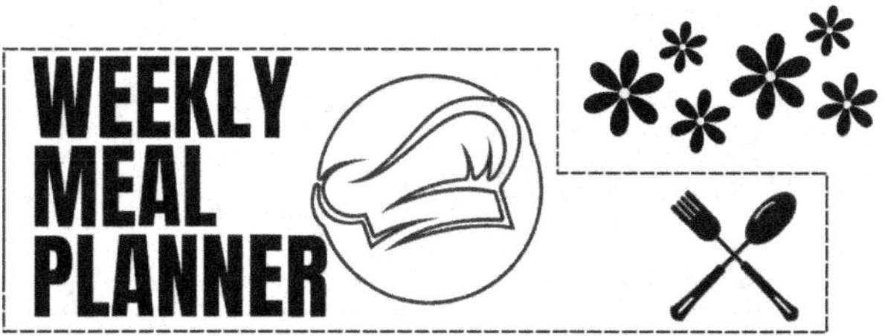

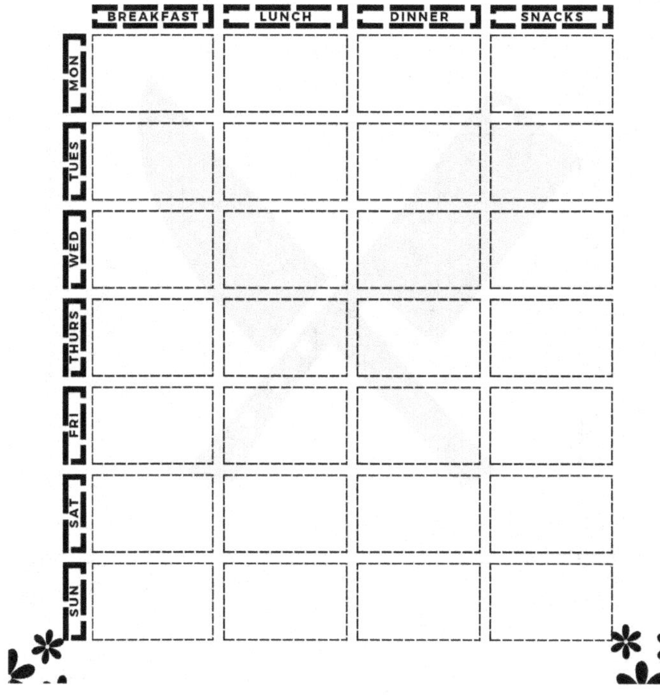

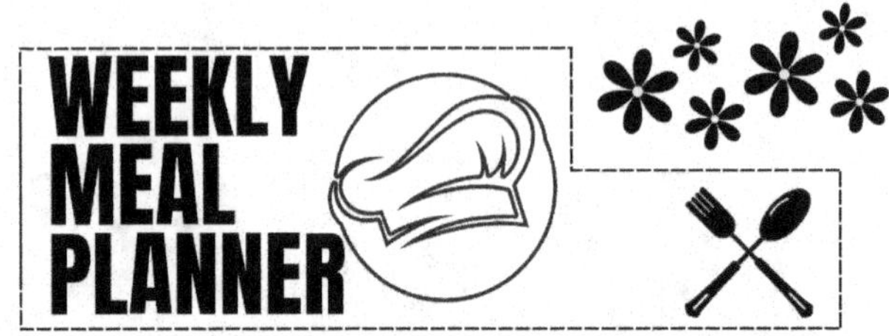

WEEKLY
MEAL
PLANNER

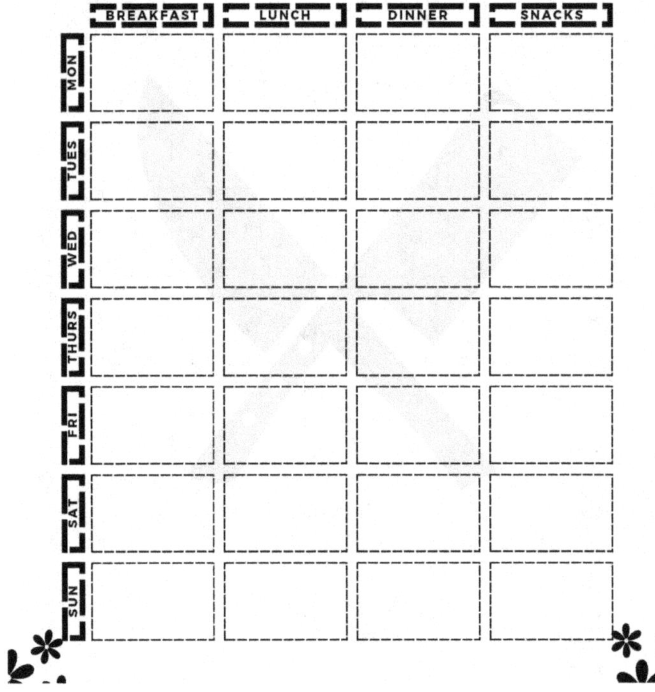

BREAKFAST
LUNCH
DINNER
SNACKS
MON
TUES
WED
THURS
FRI
SAT
SUN

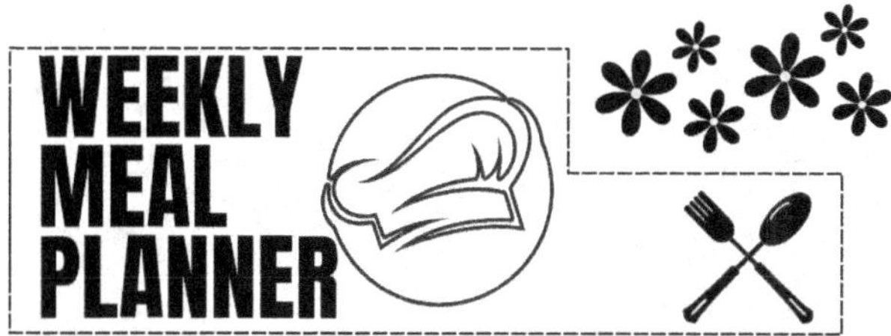

WEEKLY
MEAL
PLANNER

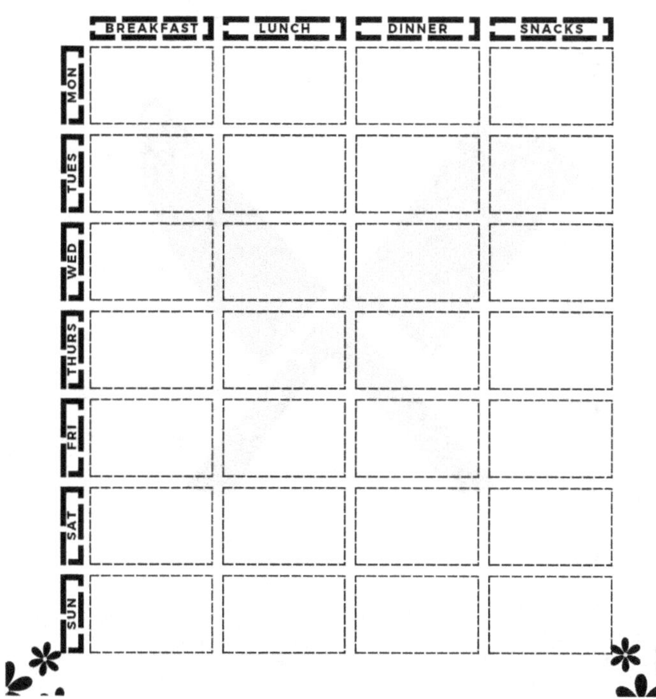

BREAKFAST
LUNCH
DINNER
SNACKS
MON
TUES
WED
THURS
FRI
SAT
SUN

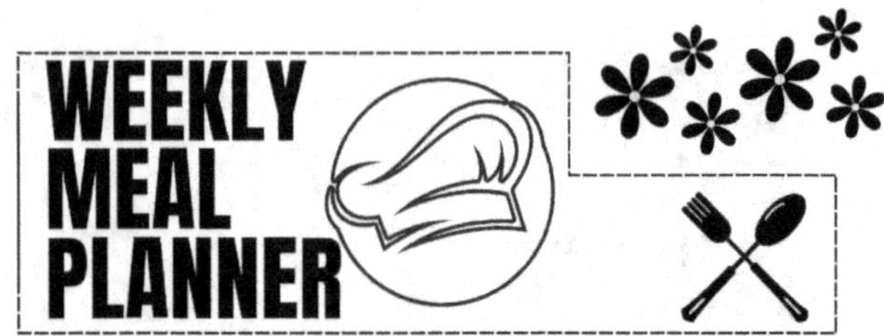

WEEKLY
MEAL
PLANNER

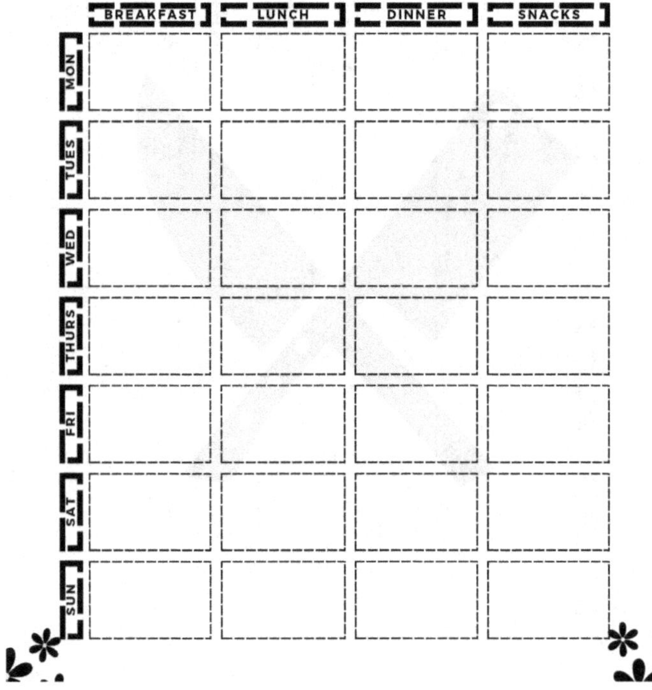

BREAKFAST
LUNCH
DINNER
SNACKS
MON
TUES
WED
THURS
FRI
SAT
SUN

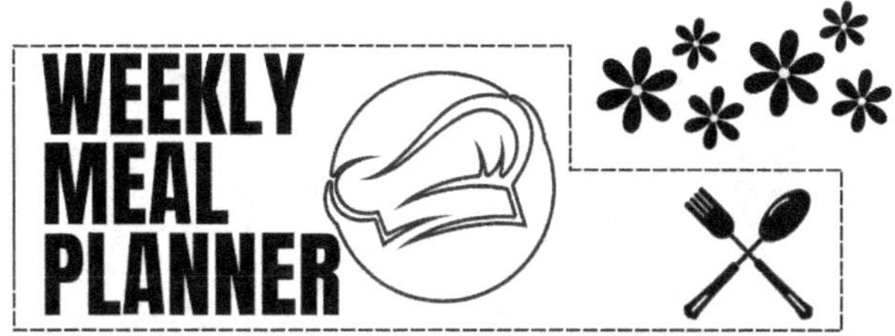

WEEKLY
MEAL
PLANNER

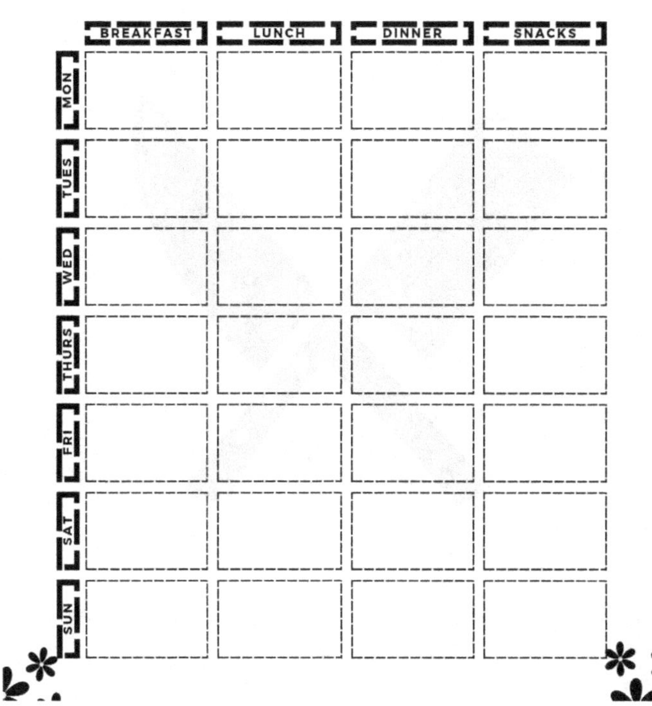

BREAKFAST
LUNCH
DINNER
SNACKS
MON
TUES
WED
THURS
FRI
SAT
SUN

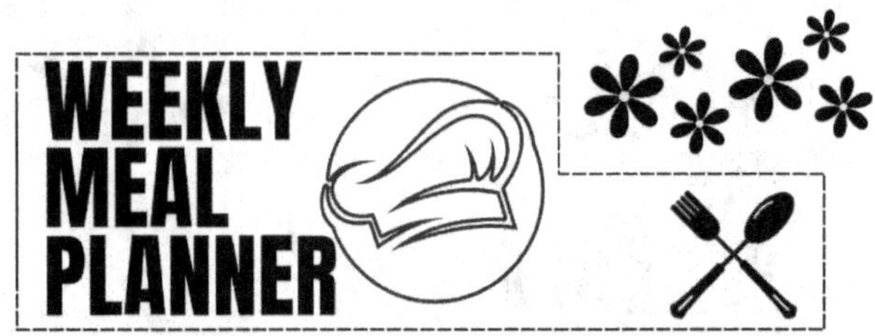

	BREAKFAST	LUNCH	DINNER	SNACKS
MON				
TUES				
WED				
THURS				
FRI				
SAT				
SUN				

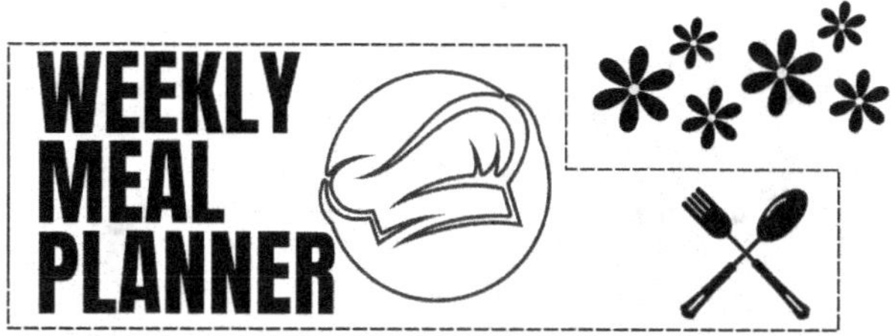

WEEKLY
MEAL
PLANNER

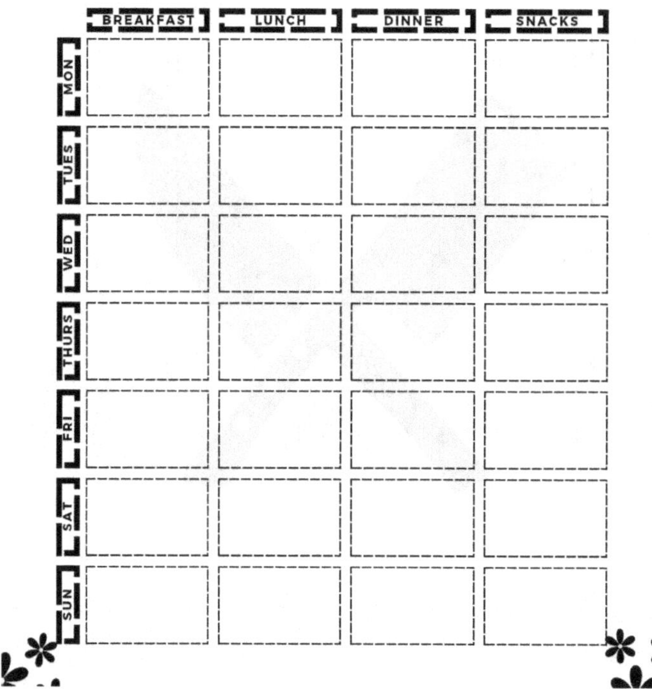

BREAKFAST
LUNCH
DINNER
SNACKS
MON
TUES
WED
THURS
FRI
SAT
SUN

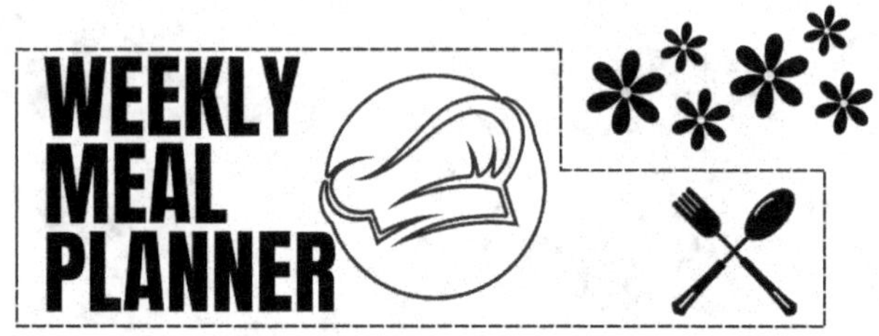

WEEKLY
MEAL
PLANNER

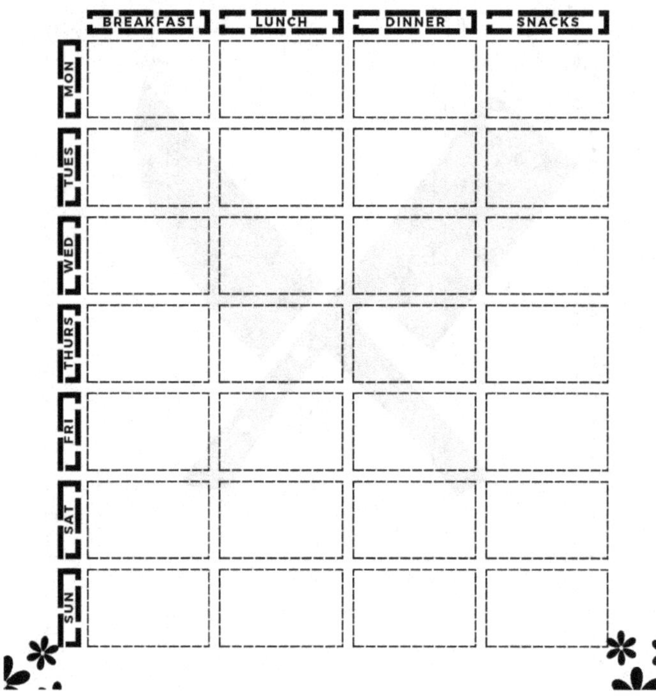

BREAKFAST
LUNCH
DINNER
SNACKS
MON
TUES
WED
THURS
FRI
SAT
SUN

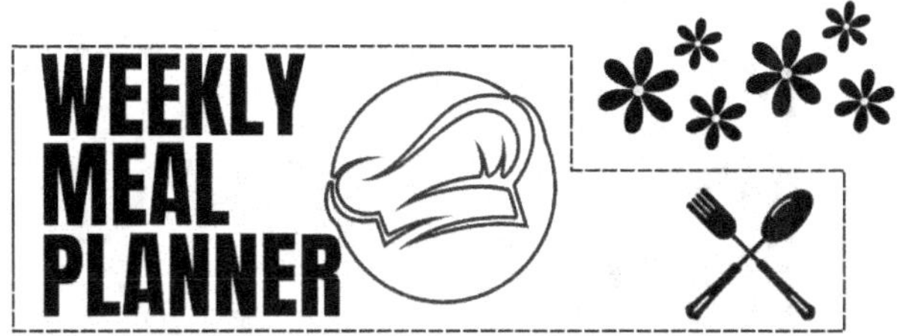

WEEKLY
MEAL
PLANNER

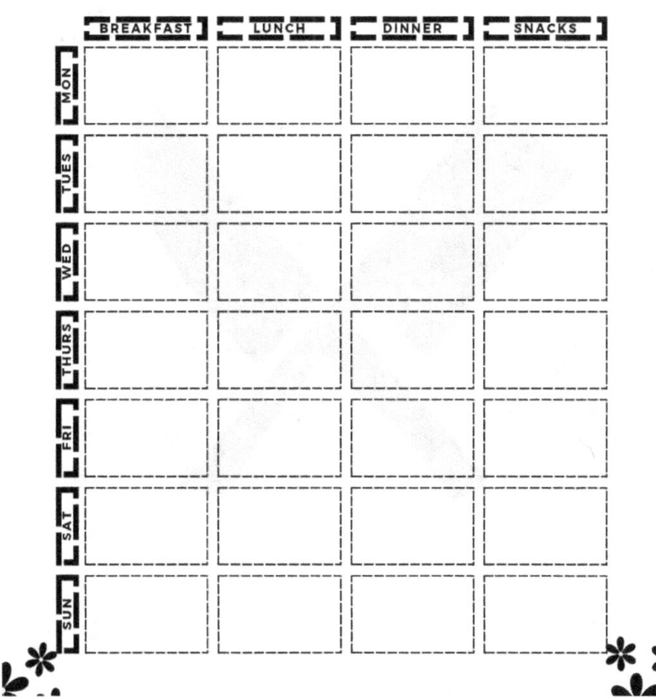

BREAKFAST
LUNCH
DINNER
SNACKS
MON
TUES
WED
THURS
FRI
SAT
SUN

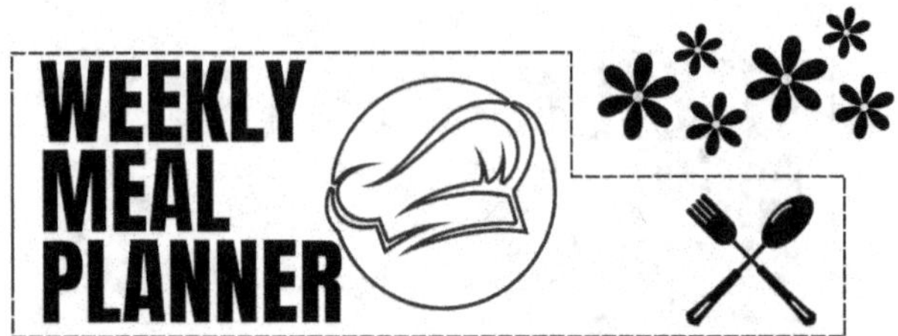

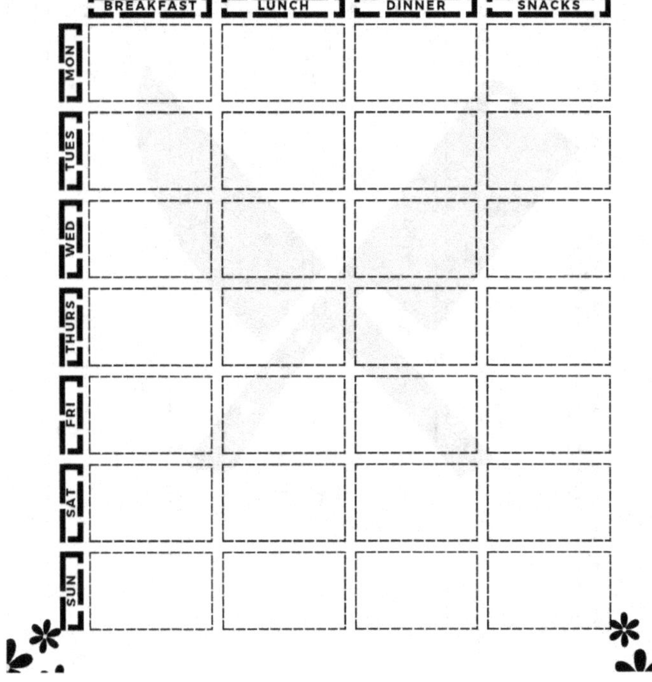

BREAKFAST
LUNCH
DINNER
SNACKS
MON
TUES
WED
THURS
FRI
SAT
SUN

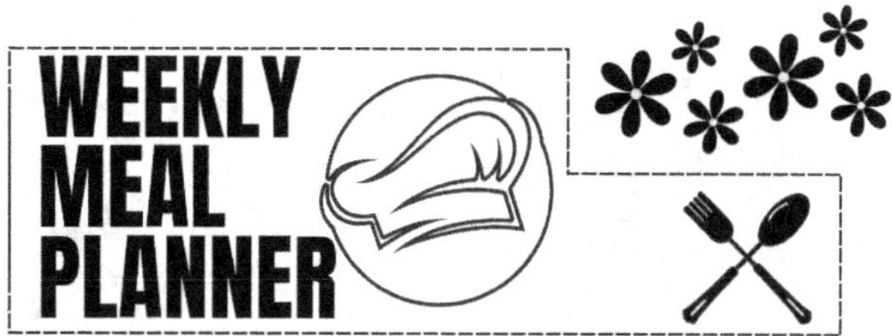

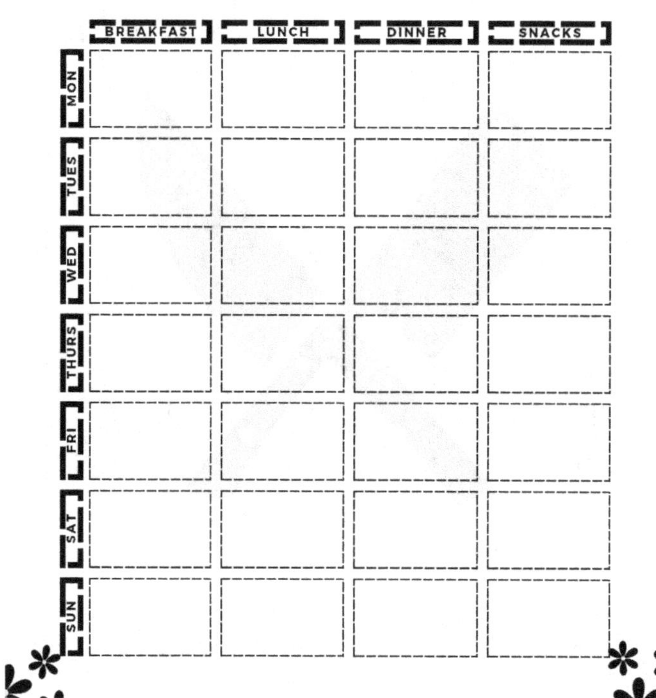

BREAKFAST
LUNCH
DINNER
SNACKS
MON
TUES
WED
THURS
FRI
SAT
SUN

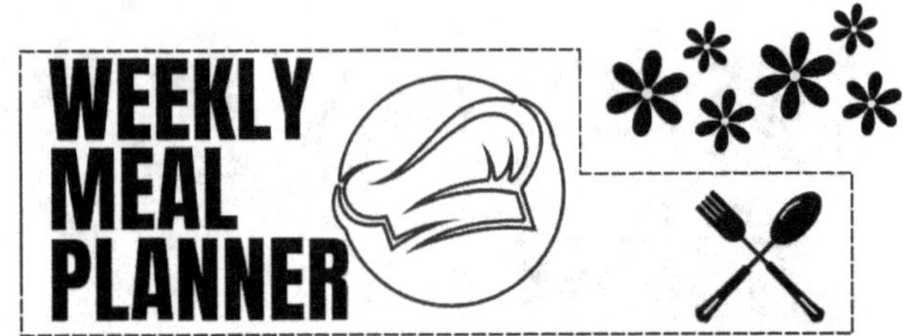

WEEKLY
MEAL
PLANNER

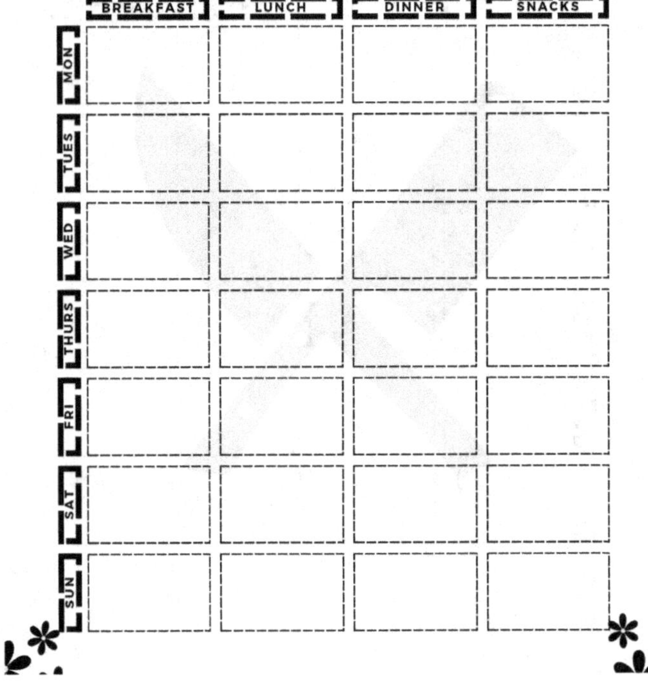

BREAKFAST
LUNCH
DINNER
SNACKS
MON
TUES
WED
THURS
FRI
SAT
SUN

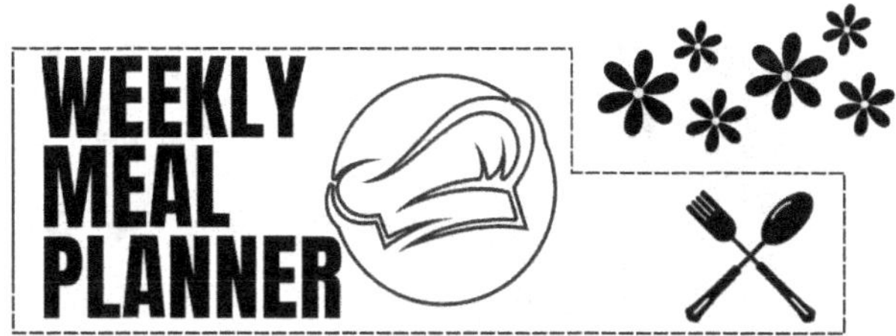

WEEKLY
MEAL
PLANNER

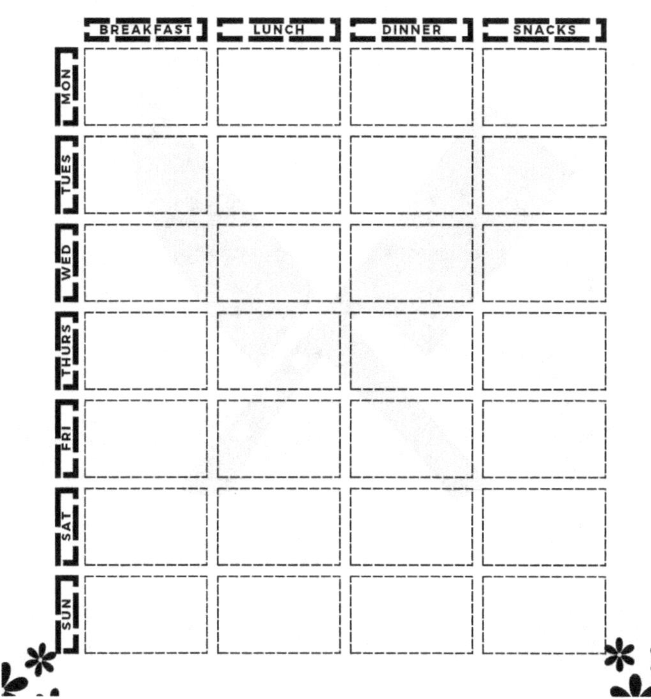

BREAKFAST
LUNCH
DINNER
SNACKS
MON
TUES
WED
THURS
FRI
SAT
SUN

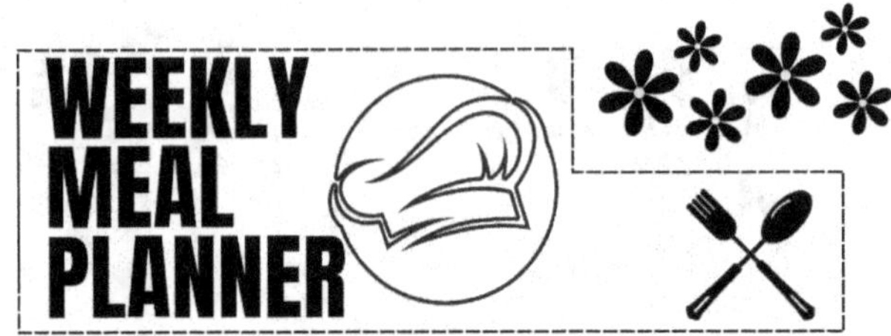

WEEKLY
MEAL
PLANNER

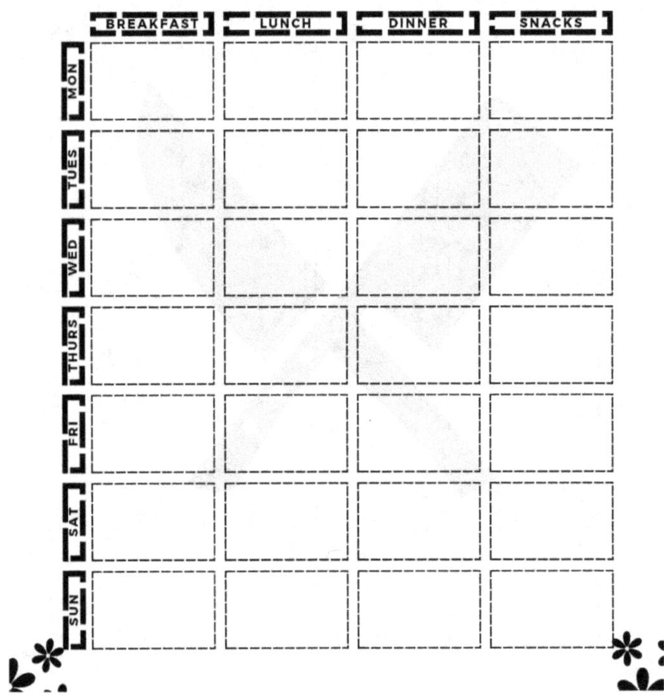

BREAKFAST
LUNCH
DINNER
SNACKS
MON
TUES
WED
THURS
FRI
SAT
SUN

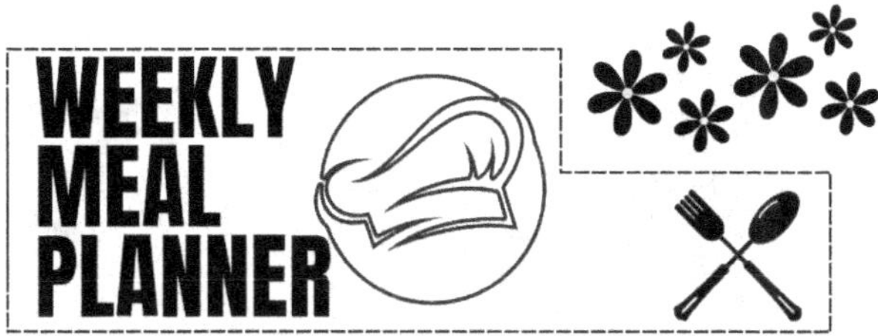
WEEKLY
MEAL
PLANNER

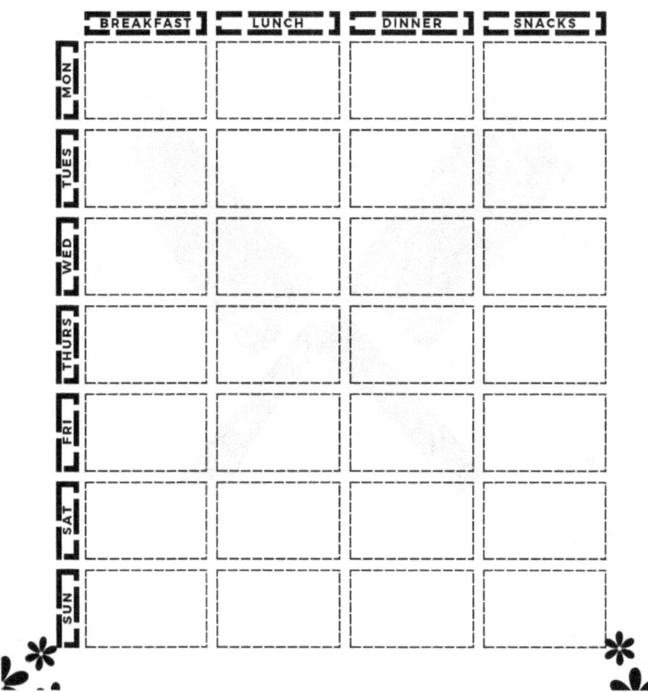
BREAKFAST
LUNCH
DINNER
SNACKS
MON
TUES
WED
THURS
FRI
SAT
SUN

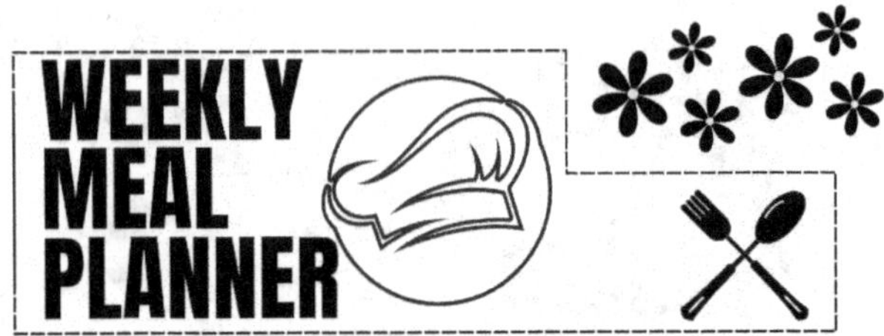

WEEKLY
MEAL
PLANNER

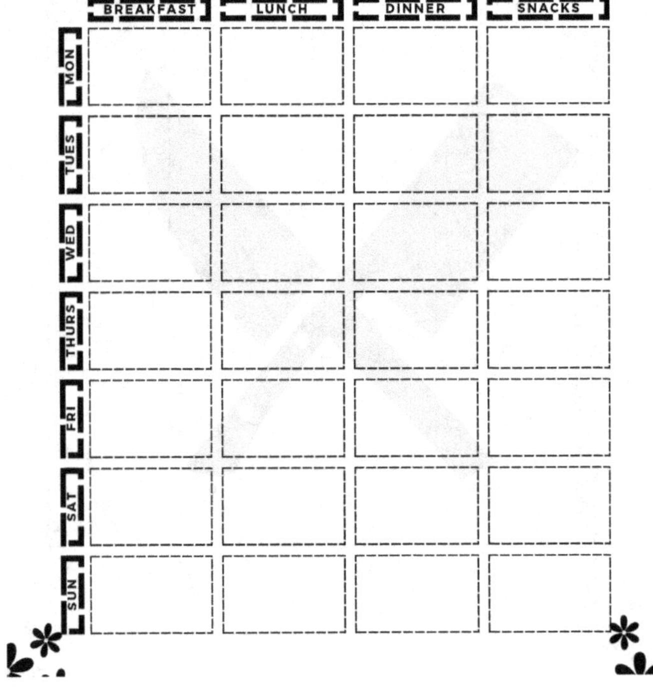

BREAKFAST
LUNCH
DINNER
SNACKS
MON
TUES
WED
THURS
FRI
SAT
SUN

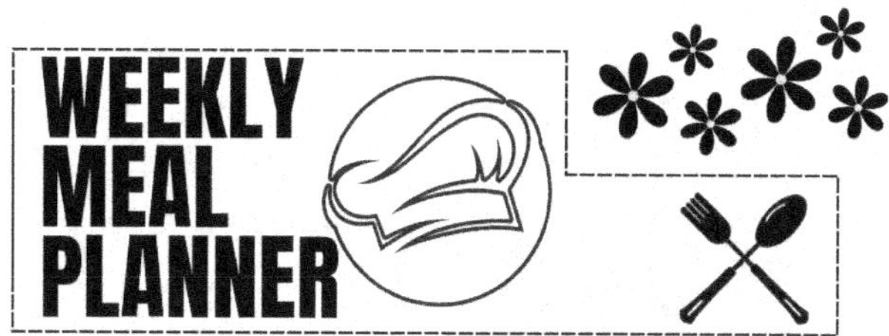

WEEKLY
MEAL
PLANNER

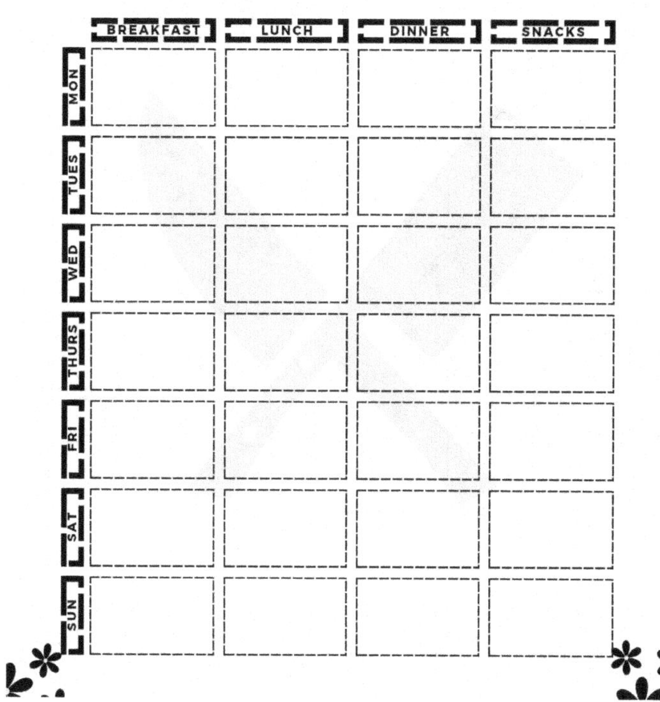

BREAKFAST
LUNCH
DINNER
SNACKS
MON
TUES
WED
THURS
FRI
SAT
SUN

WEEKLY MEAL PLANNER

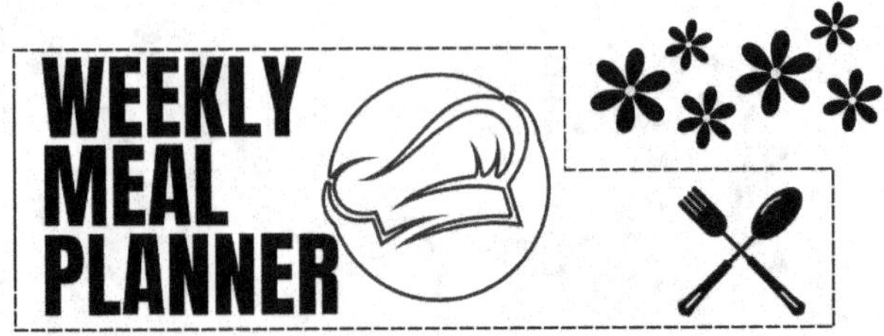

	BREAKFAST	LUNCH	DINNER	SNACKS
MON				
TUES				
WED				
THURS				
FRI				
SAT				
SUN				

FATTY LIVER DIET COOKBOOK FOR SENIORS

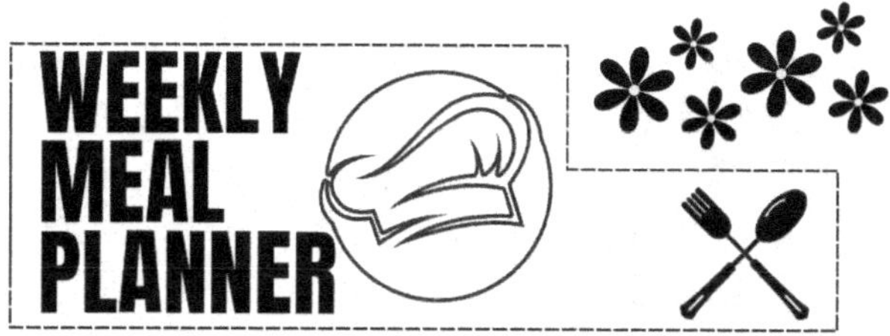

WEEKLY
MEAL
PLANNER

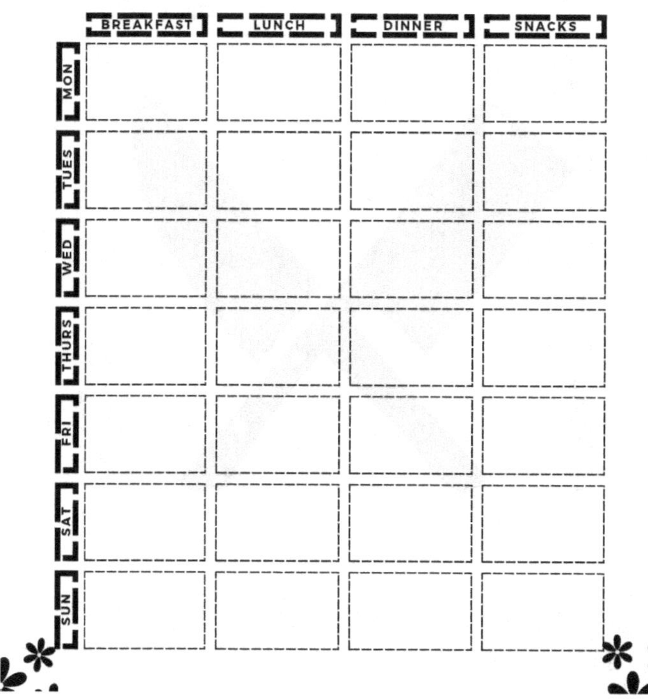

BREAKFAST
LUNCH
DINNER
SNACKS
MON
TUES
WED
THURS
FRI
SAT
SUN

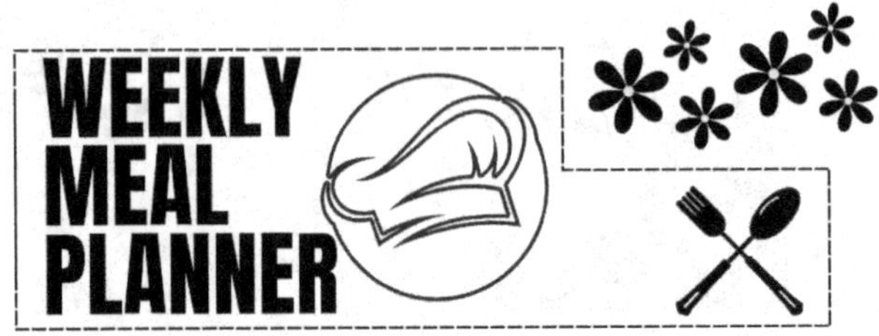

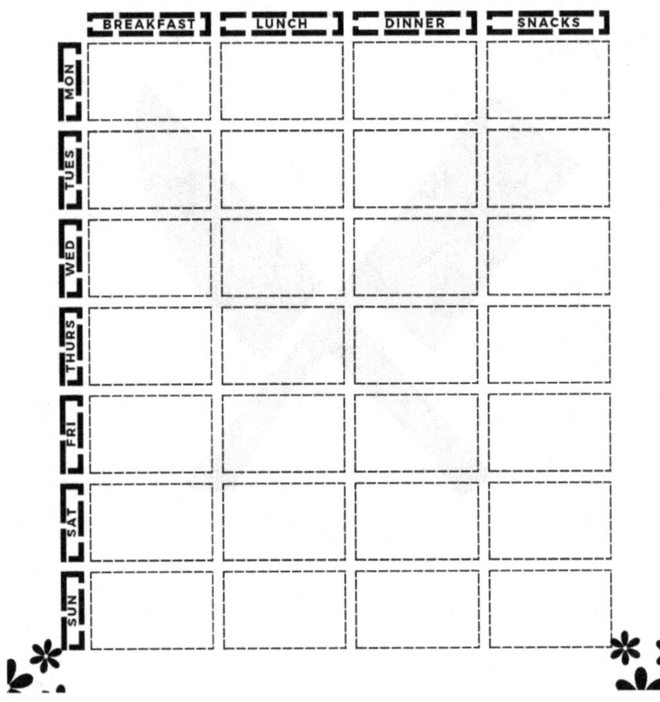

FATTY LIVER DIET COOKBOOK FOR SENIORS

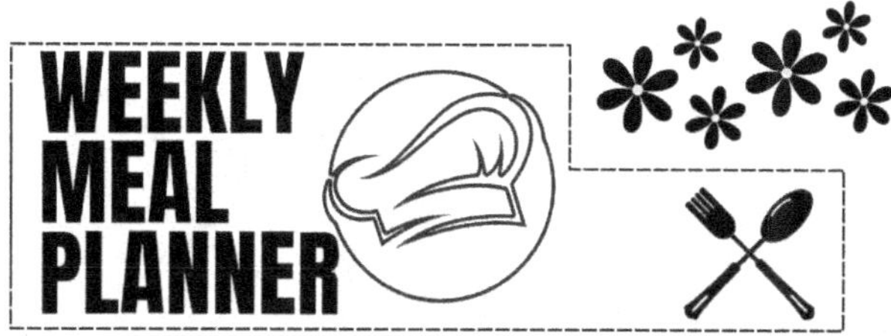

WEEKLY
MEAL
PLANNER

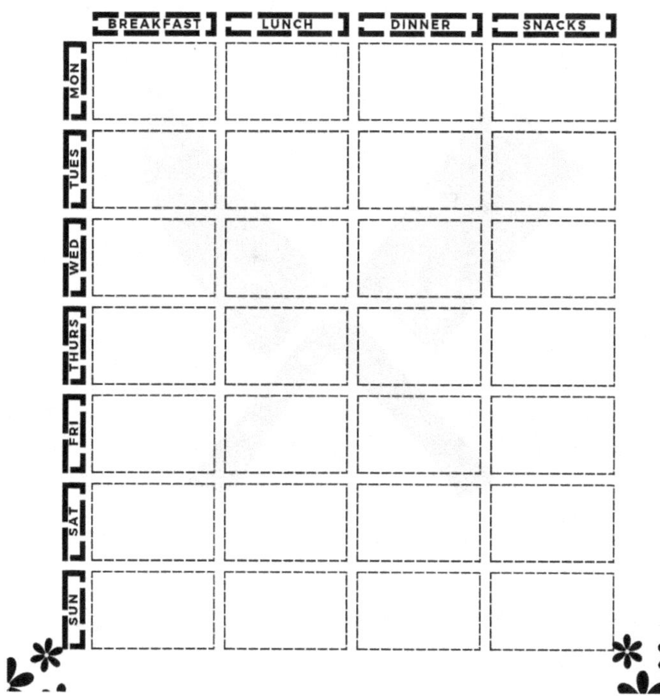

BREAKFAST
LUNCH
DINNER
SNACKS
MON
TUES
WED
THURS
FRI
SAT
SUN